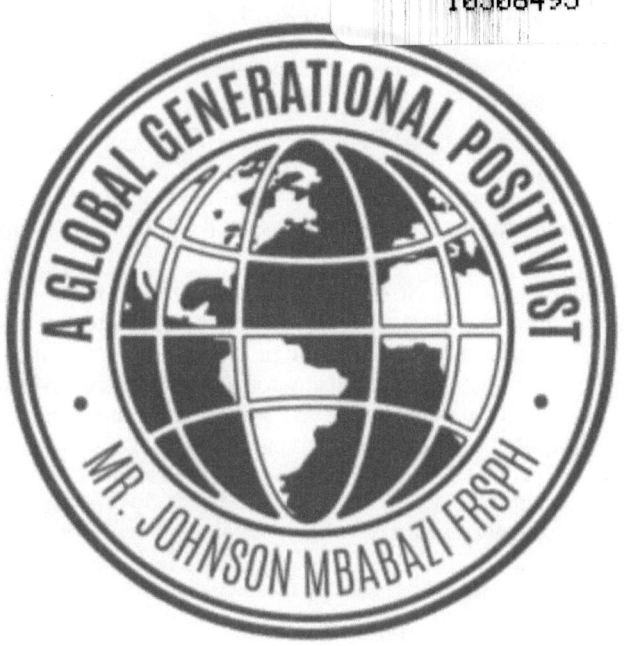

Clinical advice, deeper understanding, guidance and management of lymphoma cancer

Johnson Mbabazi FRSPH

Published by New Generation Publishing in 2021

Copyright © Johnson Mbabazi FRSPH 2021

First Edition

The author asserts the moral right under the Copyright, Designs and Patents Act 1988 to be identified as the author of this work.

All Rights reserved. No part of this publication may be reproduced, stored in a retrieval system or transmitted, in any form or by any means without the prior consent of the author, nor be otherwise circulated in any form of binding or cover other than that which it is published and without a similar condition being imposed on the subsequent purchaser.

ISBN 978-1-80031-247-0

www.newgeneration-publishing.com

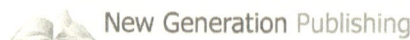

Contents
Glossary

A	1
B	3
C	5
D	8
E	9
F	10
G	11
H	12
I	14
L	15
M	17
N	18
O	19
P	20
R	23
S	24
T	26
V	27
W	28
X	28

1 Causes of lymphoma 29
2 The lymphatic system..29
2.1 What is the lymphatic system and what does it do? 29
3 The immune system...38
3.1 What is the immune system?................................38
3.2 Physical barriers 39
3.2.1 Phagocytes 40
3.2.2 Lymphocytes and antibodies 40
3.2.3 Immune cells and proteins that help lymphocytes 42
3.3 What can go wrong with the immune system?....43
3.3.1 The immune system and cancer...................43
3.4 What is cancer?...44
4 Lymphoma and the immune system.......................44
4.1 How does lymphoma affect the immune system?...44
4.2 How does treatment for lymphoma affect the immune system? 45
4.2.1 Effects of treatment on your immune system..45
4.2.2 Other ways treatment can affect your immune system 46

	4.3	The immune system after treatment 47
	4.4	Using the immune system to treat lymphoma 49
5		**Coping with symptoms of lymphoma 68**
	5.1	Coping with common symptoms of lymphoma .. 69
	5.2	Coping with swollen lymph nodes 69
	5.3	Coping with fatigue 70
	5.4	Coping with weight loss 70
	5.5	Coping with night sweats 71
	5.6	Coping with itching 72
	5.6.1	General tips 73
	5.6.2	Bathing and showering 74
	5.6.3	Clothes 75
	5.7	Coping with pain 75
	5.8	Coping with skin symptoms 76
	5.8.1	Skin care 77
	5.8.2	Healthcare 77
	5.8.3	Clothing 77
	5.8.4	Lifestyle 77
	5.9	Coping with your emotions 78
6		**Tests, diagnosis and staging 78**
	6.1	Getting a referral for tests 78
	6.2	Blood tests 79
	6.3	X-ray, CT, MRI, and PET scans 79

7 Scans: X-ray, CT, PET and MRI 80

7.1 Overview of scans 80

7.1.1 What is a scan? 80
7.1.2 What are scans used for? 80
7.1.3 Why are there different types of scans? 80
7.1.4 What is a contrast agent? 81
7.1.5 Are scans safe? 81

7.2 What is an X-ray scan? 81

7.3 What is the process for having an X-ray scan? ... 83

7.3.1 How should I prepare? 83
7.3.2 What happens during the procedure? 83
7.3.3 What happens after the procedure? 84

7.4 What is a computed tomography (CT) scan? 84

7.5 What is the process for having a CT scan? 86

7.5.1 How should I prepare? 86
7.5.2 What happens during the procedure? 87
7.5.3 What happens after the procedure? 87

7.6 What is a positron-emission tomography (PET) scan? 88

7.7 What is the process for having a PET scan? 90

7.7.1 How should I prepare? 91
7.7.2 What happens during the procedure? 92

7.8 What is a magnetic resonance imaging (MRI) scan? 93

7.9 What is the process for having an MRI scan?.....95

    7.9.1 How should I prepare?..................95

    7.9.2 What happens during the procedure? 96

    7.9.3 What happens after the procedure? 97

7.10 Frequently asked questions about scans...............97

    7.10.1 Can I have a scan if I am pregnant or breastfeeding? 97

    7.10.2 Are scans painful? 99

    7.10.3 Do scans use radiation? 99

    7.10.4 Will I be radioactive after a scan? 99

    7.10.5 Are there any side effects of having a contrast agent? 100

    7.10.6 When will I get the results? 101

    7.10.7 I feel anxious about having the scan – what can I do? 101

7.11 Ultrasound scan 102

8 Ultrasound scan 102

8.1 What is an ultrasound scan? 102

8.2 What is the process for having an ultrasound scan? 104

    8.2.1 How do I prepare for an ultrasound scan?........ 104

    8.2.2 What happens during the procedure? 104

    External ultrasound scan 105

Internal ultrasound scan..105

   8.2.3   What happens after the procedure?............106

 8.3   Frequently asked questions about ultrasound scans 106

   8.3.1   Do I need to fast (not eat or drink) on the day of the scan?..106

   8.3.2   Is it Okay to take prescription medication before the scan?..106

   8.3.3   Will I be closed in during the scan?...........106

   8.3.4   When will I get the results? 106

   8.3.5   Are ultrasound scans safe?..........................107

   8.3.6   Can I have an ultrasound scan if I am pregnant or breastfeeding? 107

 8.4   What if I feel anxious about having the scan?...107

 8.5   Biopsy..108

9   **Biopsy 108**

 9.1   What is a biopsy? 108

 9.2   Why might I need a biopsy?...............................110

 9.3   What are the different types of biopsy?.............111

   9.3.1   Excision biopsy..111

   9.3.2   Incisional biopsy 112

   9.3.3   Core needle biopsy 112

   9.3.4   Laparoscopic (keyhole) biopsy...................113

 9.4   How should I care for the biopsied area? 114

- 9.4.1 How long does it take to recover after a biopsy? 114
- 9.5 How long does it take for results to come back? 115
- 9.6 Will I need further tests? 115
  - 9.6.1 What other tests might I have? 116
    - Fine needle aspiration cytology 116
    - Endobronchial ultrasound-guided fine needle aspiration 116
- 9.7 Here are the answers to some frequently asked questions and concerns about biopsies. 117
  - 9.7.1 Is a biopsy painful? 117
  - 9.7.2 Can removing a lymph node affect my immunity? 117
  - 9.7.3 Does removing an affected lymph node remove the lymphoma? 117
- 9.8 Bone marrow tests 118

10 Bone marrow biopsy 118
- 10.1 What is bone marrow? 118
- 10.2 What is a bone marrow biopsy? 119
- 10.3 Who might need a bone marrow biopsy? 120
- 10.4 What is the process for having a bone marrow biopsy? 120
  - 10.4.1 How should I prepare? 121
  - 10.4.2 What happens during the procedure? 121

  10.4.3 What happens after the procedure?............123

 10.5 Is a bone marrow biopsy safe? 124

 10.6 When will I get the results? 124

 10.7 Lumbar puncture 125

11 Lumbar puncture 125

 11.1 What is a lumbar puncture? 125

 11.2 Who might need a lumbar puncture? 126

 11.3 What is the process for having a lumbar puncture? 127

  11.3.1 How should I prepare? 127

  11.3.2 What happens during the procedure? 127

  11.3.3 What happens after the procedure?............129

 11.4 Is a lumbar puncture safe? 129

 11.5 When will I get the results? 130

 11.6 Waiting for your results 130

12 Treatment for lymphoma 146

 12.1 How do my medical team decide what treatment I need? 146

 12.2 What do I need to know about my treatment? ...147

 12.3 Where can I find more information about treatment for lymphoma? 148

13 Active monitoring (watch and wait) 149

 13.1 What is active monitoring? 149

 13.2 Why is active monitoring done? 150

13.3 Who might have active monitoring? 151
   13.3.1 Are there any other options? 152
13.4 What happens on active monitoring? 153
13.5 When does treatment start? 154
13.6 Living with active monitoring 155
   13.6.1 What can I do to help myself? 156

14 Chemotherapy 157
   14.1.1 What is the aim of chemotherapy? 157
   14.1.2 How often do I have treatment and how long does a course last? 158
   14.1.3 How is chemotherapy given? 158
   14.1.4 Is chemotherapy painful? 158
   14.1.5 What are the side effects of chemotherapy? 158
14.2 What is chemotherapy? 159
14.3 How does chemotherapy work? 159
   14.3.1 Chemotherapy regimens (combinations of drugs) 160
14.4 Why is chemotherapy used to treat lymphoma? 160
14.5 How is chemotherapy given? 161
   14.5.1 Oral chemotherapy 161
   14.5.2 Intravenous (IV) chemotherapy 161
   IV chemotherapy through a cannula 161

IV given through a central venous catheter ('line') 163

Intrathecal chemotherapy 164

Subcutaneous chemotherapy 165

14.6 What side effects might I have? 165

14.6.1 Other possible side effects 167

14.7 What late effects might I have? 168

14.7.1 Effects on fertility 168

14.7.2 Second cancers 168

14.8 How will I be followed-up after treatment? 169

14.9 Frequently asked questions 169

14.9.1 Will I have other treatments together with my chemotherapy? 170

14.9.2 Why can't surgery cure my lymphoma? 170

14.9.3 How can I reduce my risk of infection while I'm having treatment? 171

14.9.4 How long do chemotherapy drugs stay in your body? 171

14.9.5 Can I drink alcohol? 171

14.9.6 Can I smoke? 172

14.9.7 Is it safe to exercise? 172

14.9.8 Am I likely to lose my hair? 172

14.9.9 Is it safe to have a massage? 173

14.9.10 Could complementary therapies help me?....... 173

14.9.11 Can I carry on working? 173

14.9.12 Can I see friends and family? 174

14.9.13 Can I have a flu vaccination? 174

14.9.14 Are there any restrictions in what I can eat? ... .174

14.9.15 Can I go out in public? 175

14.9.16 Can I have sex?... 175

14.9.17 When can I get pregnant after my treatment?.. 175

14.9.18 Can I breastfeed while I am having treatment? 176

14.9.19 Can I go on holiday when I am having chemotherapy? 176

15 Chemotherapy regimens for lymphoma 176

15.1 What is a chemotherapy regimen? 176

15.2 Common chemotherapy regimens for lymphoma... 177

15.2.1 Acronyms for chemotherapy regimens sometimes used to treat lymphoma 178

15.3 Which chemotherapy regimen might I have? ... 180

15.4 Side effects of chemotherapy regimens 180

16 CNS prophylaxis.. 181

16.1 What is CNS prophylaxis? 181

 16.2 Who might need CNS prophylaxis?...................184

 16.3 How is CNS prophylaxis given? 186

  16.3.1 Intrathecal chemotherapy............................186

  Intravenous chemotherapy 187

17 Radiotherapy 188

 17.1 Quick overview 188

  17.1.1 What is the aim of radiotherapy?...............188

  17.1.2 How often will I have treatment and how long does it take?...188

  17.1.3 Is radiotherapy painful? 189

  17.1.4 What are the side effects of radiotherapy? ......
....189

 17.2 What is radiotherapy?..189

  17.2.1 How does radiotherapy work? 189

 17.3 Radiotherapy for lymphoma...............................190

  17.3.1 Radiotherapy to cure lymphoma (curative radiotherapy) 190

  17.3.2 Radiotherapy to control symptoms of lymphoma (palliative radiotherapy).........................191

  17.3.3 When will I have radiotherapy?..................191

  17.3.4 Which types of lymphoma does radiotherapy treat? 191

  Radiotherapy for Hodgkin lymphoma.................191

  Radiotherapy for non-Hodgkin lymphoma 192

17.4 What types of radiotherapy are there?...............192

    17.4.1 Total body irradiation (TBI).......................195

    17.4.2 Total skin electron radiotherapy (TSET)...196

17.5 Where will I have radiotherapy? 196

17.6 How much radiotherapy will I need? 196

17.7 How is radiotherapy planned?...........................197

    17.7.1 How your radiotherapy is planned.............198

    17.7.2 Treatment shell or mask 199

17.8 What happens during a radiotherapy session? ..200

    17.8.1 Setting up...200

    17.8.2 Having your radiotherapy..........................200

17.9 What side effects might I have? 201

    17.9.1 Fatigue 202

    17.9.2 Sore skin 202

    17.9.3 Sore mouth and throat/discomfort swallowing (mucositis)..203

    17.9.4 Nausea (feeling sick) 203

    17.9.5 Diarrhoea 204

    17.9.6 Hair loss..204

17.10 What late effects might I have?.......................204

    17.10.1 Dental problems...205

    17.10.2 Eye problems 205

    17.10.3 Heart problems 205

17.10.4 Mouth dryness 205

17.10.5 Reduced fertility 205

17.10.6 Risk of developing a cancer related to radiotherapy 206

17.10.7 Lung problems 206

17.10.8 Thyroid problems 206

17.11 How will I be followed-up after treatment? 207

17.12 Frequently asked questions 208

17.12.1 Will radiotherapy make me radioactive? ... 208

17.12.2 Can I take someone into the room with me when I have radiotherapy? 208

17.12.3 Can I call for attention during treatment if I need to? 208

17.12.4 Is it safe to have radiotherapy if I have a pacemaker (cardiac rhythm device)? 208

17.12.5 Is it safe to have radiotherapy while I am pregnant? 209

17.12.6 Can I breastfeed if I am having radiotherapy?. 209

18 Antibody therapy for lymphoma (including rituximab) 209

18.1 What are antibodies? 209

18.2 What is antibody therapy? 210

18.3 How does antibody therapy work? 211

19 Rituximab for lymphoma 212

- 19.1 What is rituximab? 213
- 19.2 Who can have it? 214
  - 19.2.1 Is it available on the NHS in the UK? 214
- 19.3 Benefits..214
- 19.4 How is it given?..217
  - 19.4.1 Intravenous infusion 218
  - 19.4.2 Subcutaneous injection 218
- 19.5 Possible side effects 218
  - 19.5.1 Other severe side effects.............................221
    - Severe infusion-related reactions 221
    - Increased risk of infection 222
    - Other low blood counts 222
  - 19.5.2 Are there any side effects with rituximab by subcutaneous injection? 223
- 19.6 Precautions 223

20 Newer antibodies against...................................224
- 20.1 Antibodies targeting CD20....................................224
- 20.2 Ofatumumab (Arzerra®)..225
  - 20.2.1 Who can have it? 225
  - 20.2.2 Benefits..226
  - 20.2.3 How is it given?..227
  - 20.2.4 Possible side effects....................................227
  - 20.2.5 Are there any other precautions?................229

- 20.3 Obinutuzumab (Gazyvaro®) 230
  - 20.3.1 Who can have it? 230
  - 20.3.2 Benefits 232
  - 20.3.3 How is it given? 233
  - 20.3.4 Possible side effects 234
  - 20.3.5 Are there any other precautions? 235

21 Targeted drugs for lymphoma 236
- 21.1 What are targeted drugs? 236
- 21.2 Who can have targeted drugs? 237
- 21.3 What targeted drugs are approved for lymphoma? 238
- 21.4 Lymphoma research and drugs in development 240

22 Lymphoma drug development, approval and funding 240
- 22.1 Drug development 240
  - 22.1.1 Pre-discovery and drug discovery 242
  - 22.1.2 Pre-clinical tests 242
  - 22.1.3 Clinical trials 242
- 22.2 Drug approval 243
  - 22.2.1 Who approves new drugs? 243
- 22.3 Funding 244
  - 22.3.1 How can I find out if a drug is available for me? 244

- 22.3.2 What is the Cancer Drugs Fund?................245
- 22.3.3 What is the Early Access to Medicines Scheme? 246
- 22.3.4 How can I access drugs that are not funded?... 247

23 Brentuximab vedotin 247
- 23.1 What is brentuximab vedotin?..........................247
- 23.2 Who can have it? 248
  - 23.2.1 Is it available on the NHS in the UK? 249
  - 23.2.2 What can I do if brentuximab vedotin isn't funded for me? 250
- 23.3 Benefits...250
  - 23.3.1 Benefits in classical Hodgkin lymphoma 250
  - 23.3.2 Benefits in systemic ALCL 251
  - 23.3.3 Benefits in CTCL..251
- 23.4 How is it given?..252
- 23.5 Possible side effects 252
- 23.6 Precautions 254

24 CAR T cells 255
- 24.1 What are CAR T cells?.....................................255
  - 24.1.1 The parts of a CAR T cell...........................256
- 24.2 Who can have them? 257

  24.2.1 Are they available on the NHS in the UK?......
....258

 24.3 Benefits..258
  24.3.1 Benefits of axicabtagene ciloleucel 258
  24.3.2 Benefits of tisagenlecleucel 259
 24.4 How are they given?..259
  24.4.1 Step 1: Lymphocyte collection 260
  24.4.2 Step 2: Manufacture of CAR T cells 260
  24.4.3 Step 3: Chemotherapy................................261
  24.4.4 Step 4: CAR T-cell infusion 261
 24.5 Possible side effects...262
  24.5.1 Cytokine release syndrome........................263
  24.5.2 Other immune system side effects..............264
  24.5.3 Nervous system problems..........................264
 24.6 Precautions 265

25 Checkpoint inhibitors 265
 25.1 What are checkpoint inhibitors?.........................266
 25.2 Who can have them? 268
  25.2.1 Are they available on the NHS in the UK?......
....269

 25.3 Benefits..270
  25.3.1 Benefits of nivolumab................................270
  25.3.2 Benefits of pembrolizumab........................270
 25.4 How are they given?..270

- 25.5 Possible side effects 271
- 25.6 Precautions 272

26 Ibrutinib 273
- 26.1 What is ibrutinib? 273
- 26.2 Who can have ibrutinib? 274
  - 26.2.1 Is it available on the NHS in the UK? 275
- 26.3 Benefits 276
  - 26.3.1 Benefits in mantle cell lymphoma 276
  - 26.3.2 Benefits in chronic lymphocytic leukaemia (CLL) 276
  - 26.3.3 Benefits in Waldenström's macroglobulinaemia (WM) 277
- 26.4 How is it given? 278
  - 26.4.1 When is ibrutinib given? 278
  - 26.4.2 Will I need any special tests while I am taking ibrutinib? 278
- 26.5 Possible side effects 279
  - 26.5.1 Effects on blood 280
  - 26.5.2 Bleeding problems 280
  - 26.5.3 Infections 281
  - 26.5.4 Heart problems 282
- 26.6 Who can't have ibrutinib? 282
- 26.7 Precautions 284

27 Idelalisib 285

27.1 What is idelalisib? 285
27.2 Who can have it? 286
    27.2.1 Is it available on the NHS in the UK? 286
27.3 Benefits..287
    27.3.1 Benefits in CLL/SLL 287
    27.3.2 Benefits in follicular lymphoma 288
27.4 How is it given?...288
27.5 Possible side effects..289
27.6 Precautions 291

28 Venetoclax 292
28.1 What is venetoclax?..292
28.2 Who can have it? 292
    28.2.1 Is it available on the NHS in the UK? 293
28.3 Benefits..294
28.4 How is it given?...294
28.5 Possible side effects..295
28.6 Precautions 296

29 Other targeted drugs for lymphoma 298
29.1 Types of targeted drugs 298
29.2 Radioimmunotherapy 298
    29.2.1 Zevalin® (90Y-ibritumomab tiuxetan)......298
29.3 Cell signal blockers 299
    29.3.1 Temsirolimus (Torisel®) 300

29.4 Proteasome inhibitors 300
    29.4.1 Bortezomib (Bortezomib Accord or Velcade®) 301
29.5 Immunomodulators 302
    29.5.1 Lenalidomide (Revlimid®) 302

30 Side effects of lymphoma treatment 303
    30.1 What are side effects of treatment? 303
    30.2 What are the most common side effects of lymphoma treatments? 304
        30.2.1 Side effects of chemotherapy 305
        30.2.2 Side effects of radiotherapy 306
        30.2.3 Side effects of other treatments for lymphoma 306
    30.3 What should you do if you have side effects? ... 306

31 Late effects of lymphoma treatment 307
    31.1 What are late effects? 307
        31.1.1 How to find out more about the risks of treatment 308
    31.2 Who is at increased risk of late effects? 309
    31.3 What are the potential late effects of lymphoma treatment? 310
    31.4 What are the potential late effects of chemotherapy? 310
        31.4.1 Second cancers 310
        31.4.2 Heart disease 312

	31.4.3	Lung problems 312
	31.4.4	Other late effects of chemotherapy 313
	31.4.5	Second cancers 314
	31.4.6	Heart disease and stroke 316
	31.4.7	Thyroid problems 317
	31.4.8	Effects on growth 318
	31.4.9	Other late effects of radiotherapy 318

31.5 What are the potential late effects of newer, targeted treatments? 318

31.6 How can I reduce the risk of late effects? 319

    31.6.1 Be aware of your risks – look out for symptoms 319

    31.6.2 Monitor your health to find problems early 319

    31.6.3 Follow a healthy lifestyle – give yourself the best chance of a healthy future 320

    31.6.4 Research into reducing the risk of late effects. 320

32 Living with lymphoma 321

  32.1 Staying healthy 321

  32.2 Feelings 322

  32.3 Everyday life 322

33 Self-management and remote monitoring 323

  33.1 Self-management 323

33.2 Self-management support 323
    33.2.1 Why is self-management support used? 324
    33.2.2 Who is self-management support for? 324
    33.2.3 How does self-management support work? 325
33.3 Remote monitoring 326
    33.3.1 Why is remote monitoring used? 326
    33.3.2 Who is remote monitoring for? 327
    33.3.3 How does remote monitoring work? 328
33.4 When to book an appointment 329
33.5 Life on self-management and remote monitoring ... 330

34 Lymphoma and the end of life 331

34.1 How do I know when to end active treatment? 331
    34.1.1 Is further treatment likely to work? 331
    34.1.2 What are the risks of further active treatment? 332
34.2 Can I enter a clinical trial? 332
34.3 How do I tell friends and family I'm no longer receiving active treatment? 333
34.4 How much time do I have left to live? 334
34.5 How does lymphoma lead to the end of life? 334
    34.5.1 Bone marrow failure 334

- 34.5.2 Chemical imbalance ... 335
- 34.5.3 Involvement of other organs ... 336
- 34.5.4 Hyperviscosity (thickness of blood) ... 337
- 34.5.5 Inability to close your eyes ... 338
- 34.6 What symptoms might I have as I approach the end of life? ... 338
  - 34.6.1 Itching and sweats ... 338
  - 34.6.2 Weight loss ... 338
  - 34.6.3 Loss of appetite ... 338
  - 34.6.4 Fatigue and drowsiness ... 339
  - 34.6.5 Shortness of breath ... 340
  - 34.6.6 Confusion and agitation ... 340
  - 34.6.7 Circulation ... 340
  - 34.6.8 Incontinence (loss of bladder and bowel control) ... 341
  - 34.6.9 Pain ... 341
  - 34.6.10 How can my medical team help me? ... 341
- 34.7 How will I feel emotionally? ... 342
  - 34.7.1 Shock ... 343
  - 34.7.2 Denial ... 343
  - 34.7.3 Anger ... 344
  - 34.7.4 Bargaining ... 344
  - 34.7.5 Grief and sadness ... 344

Acknowledgement

I want to acknowledge consultant Rick Jones a chemical pathologist and a Nobel prize winner that mentored me during my clinical placement, Consultant Cedric Abbott a his pathologist and consultant Orland Latimi. All these played a part in my scientific research career. I want to dedicate this research mainly to those who passed away or are dealing with lymphoma.

Abstract

Many patients with Lymphoma, has helped others given their scientific expertise and personal knowledge with a desire to manage lymphoma this difficult and often unsolved disease. Although with the availability of more effective treatment regimens, many people with lymphoma are living longer; in fact, almost two-thirds (63%) of people diagnosed with Non-Hodgkin lymphoma in England and Wales survive their disease for ten years or more (2010-11). Around 7 in 10 (69%) of people diagnosed with Non-Hodgkin lymphoma cancer in England and Wales survive their disease for five years or more (2010-11). Eight in ten (80%) of people/men/women diagnosed with Non-Hodgkin lymphoma cancer in England and Wales survive their disease for one year or more (2010-11). Non-Hodgkin lymphoma survival is similar in men than women. Non-Hodgkin lymphoma survival in England is highest for people diagnosed aged under 40 (2009-2013). Almost 9 in 10 people in England diagnosed with Non-Hodgkin lymphoma aged 15-39 survive their disease for five years or more, compared with more than 4 in 10 people diagnosed aged 80 and over (2009-2013). Non-Hodgkin lymphoma survival is improving and has tripled in the last 40 years in the UK. The 5-year survival rate for all people with Hodgkin lymphoma is 87%. The 5-year survival rate for stage I is 92%. The 5-year survival rate for stage II Hodgkin lymphoma is 93%. Approximately 40% of people are diagnosed with this stage. For stage III, the 5-year survival rate is 83% and for stage IV, it is almost 73%. It is important to remember that statistics on the survival rates for people with Hodgkin lymphoma are an estimate. The estimate comes from annual data based on the number of people with this cancer in the United States.

This book explains and provides the clinical insights of Lymphoma diagnosis, treatment, and end of life. It also describes the most current lymphoma classification and staging. More importantly, targeted therapies like ibrutinib and idelalisib and describes how other treatments, including radiation therapy and stem cell transplants, have been modified while others have been discontinued. The book also adds knowledge on the new developments on how to manage this particular type of cancer. The book includes suggestions for further reading, including the latest material available online. I highly recommend for any patient or family member seeking to understand on how to manage lymphoma to use this book. Although end of life stage can be distressing to read. I can honestly recommend it to patients, caregivers, and health professionals who will benefit from its intelligence and wisdom. It is also well guided on knowing what approach to take should be diagnosed with lymphoma.

Glossary

A

Abdomen: The middle part of the front of your body, between your chest and pelvis (the bones around your hip area)

Acute: Describes an illness or symptom that develops and progresses quickly but is short-lived

Adjuvant therapy: An additional treatment given to boost the effectiveness of the main therapy

Advanced stage: Widespread lymphoma – usually stage 3 (lymphoma on both sides of your diaphragm) or stage 4 (lymphoma that has spread to body organs outside your lymphatic system). The lymphatic system is all over the body, so it isn't unusual to find that lymphoma is widespread when it is diagnosed

Aetiology: The study of the causes of disease (sometimes used simply to mean the cause of a particular condition)

AIDS: Short for 'acquired immune deficiency syndrome', the illness caused by the human immunodeficiency virus or HIV

Alert card: A card with important information on for anyone treating you in an emergency. If you have an alert card for any reason, you should always carry it with you. Make copies in case you lose the original

Alkylating agents: Substances that interfere with the metabolism and growth of cells, so used as drugs to treat some cancers; examples are chlorambucil and cyclophosphamide

Allogeneic: Describes a transplant of donated tissue from someone else, sometimes known as an 'allograft' or 'donor transplant'

Alopecia: Hair loss; can occur as a result of some treatments for lymphoma

Anaemia: Shortage of haemoglobin (contained in red blood cells) which carries oxygen around the body in the bloodstream.

Anaesthetic: A drug that stops feeling, especially of pain: in a general anaesthetic the drugs will also make you unconscious; in a local anaesthetic the drug just numbs part of the body

Analgesic: Something (eg a drug) that abolishes or reduces pain

Anorexia: Loss of appetite, especially as a result of disease

Anthracyclines: Drugs that interfere with the DNA structure of cells, preventing them from dividing, so they are used to combat rapidly dividing cells such as cancer cells; examples are doxorubicin (Adriamycin®) and mitoxantrone.

Antibody: A specialised protein made by the B cells of the immune system; antibodies help to fight infection by attaching themselves to substances not normally found in the body (antigens), such as bacteria and foreign proteins, and attracting other parts of the immune system to dispose of the 'invader'

Antibody–drug conjugate: A treatment using a monoclonal antibody joined to a chemotherapy drug that can deliver the chemotherapy directly to the target cell

Antiemetic: Medicine that can help to reduce nausea (feeling sick) and vomiting (being sick)

Antigen: The part of a 'foreign' substance that has entered the body that is recognised by the immune system, which then stimulates a defensive response in the form of an antibody; the foreign substance is usually a protein

Antimetabolites: A group of anti-cancer drugs that join with the cell's DNA and stop it from dividing; examples include methotrexate, fluorouracil, fludarabine and gemcitabine

Apheresis: A procedure in which something is separated out, usually out of the blood; a special apparatus separates out one particular constituent of the blood (eg plasma, the liquid part of the blood, or cells such as stem cells) and returns the remainder of the blood to the circulation

Apoptosis: Process of cell suicide or 'programmed cell death', which is a normal body process to make way for new cells; can be triggered by chemotherapy drugs and irradiation

Aspirate: Sample of cells taken by suction using a needle

Autologous: Describes a transplant of a person's own tissue (eg of bone marrow or stem cells)

B

B cells / B lymphocytes: Cells of the immune system that produce antibodies

B symptoms: Three particularly significant symptoms – fevers, night sweats and unexplained weight loss – that can occur in people with lymphoma

Bacteria: Small organisms, some of which can cause disease

Benign Not cancerous (although benign lumps or conditions can still cause problems because of their size or position)

Biological therapies: Based on substances that the body makes naturally, these are anti-cancer treatments that work by affecting how the cancer cell works; examples are interferon and monoclonal antibodies

Biopsy: A sample of affected tissue that is taken to see if abnormal cells are present and to confirm a diagnosis; for people with lymphoma the commonest biopsy is a lymph node biopsy (examination of the cells and their 'architecture' or arrangement under the microscope will indicate what type of lymphoma it is)

Biosimilar: A drug designed to be very similar to a drug that is already being used (the 'reference drug'). Biosimilars must be shown to be as safe and effective as the reference drug in clinical trials before they are approved for use

Blast cell: An immature blood cell, which does not normally appear in the healthy bloodstream

Blind or blinding: means that people taking part in a clinical trial don't know what treatment they are receiving. Sometimes, the doctor doesn't know either – this is called a 'double-blind' trial

Blood–brain barrier: A barrier of cells and blood vessels that only lets certain substances reach the brain, protecting it from harmful chemicals and infections

Blood cells: The three main types of cells or cell fragments present in the blood are red cells, white cells and platelets

Blood count: A sample of blood is taken and the numbers of different cells present in the blood sample are checked using a microscope and compared with the 'normal range' of cell numbers found in healthy blood

Bone marrow: The spongy tissue in the centre of some of the large bones of the body where blood cells are made

Broviac® line: A type of central line sometimes used in children

---

C

Cancer cells: Cells that have characteristics which make them different from normal cells, for example in their genetic make-up, their ability to keep on multiplying, their failure to mature and die, their ability to grow in the wrong place in the body or spread to other parts of the body via the bloodstream or lymphatic system

Cancer drugs fund (CDF): Money currently being made available in England that pays for selected cancer drugs that could otherwise not be given to people on the NHS

Candida: A fungus that can cause an infection in the lining of the mouth (oral thrush) especially in people who have a weakened immune system

Cannula: A soft flexible tube which is inserted into the body, usually into a vein, and through which fluids and medicines can be passed into the body without the need for repeated injections

Carcinogenic: Something that can make cells become cancerous

Cardiovascular: Relating to the heart and blood vessels

Catheter: A flexible, hollow tube which can be inserted into an organ so that fluids or gases can be removed from, or administered into, the body

CD20: A protein 'marker' found on the surface of mature B cells and on the surface of certain lymphomas, which is why it is targeted by specialised anti-lymphoma treatments called monoclonal antibodies

Cell: The microscopic building block of the body; all our organs are made up of cells and although they have the same basic structure, they are specially adapted to form each part of the body

Cell signal blockers: Cells receive signals that keep them alive and make them divide. These signals are sent along 1 or more pathways. Cell signal blockers are newer drugs that block either the signal or a key part of the pathway. This can make cells die or stop them from growing

Cell surface markers: Proteins found on the surface of cells which can be used to identify particular cell types; they are labelled using letters and numbers (eg CD4, CD20, in which the 'CD' stands for 'cluster of differentiation')

Central line: A thin flexible tube which is inserted into a large vein in the chest; some types can be left in place for some months, which allows all treatments to be given and all blood tests to be taken through the one line

Central nervous system (CNS): The brain and spinal cord

Cerebrospinal fluid (CSF): The fluid which bathes the tissues of the central nervous system

Chemotherapy A form of treatment that uses drugs to damage and kill rapidly dividing cells at various stages of their cycle of development

Chemo-immunotherapy: Chemotherapy (eg CHOP) with immunotherapy (eg rituximab). The initial of the immunotherapy drug is usually added to the abbreviation for the chemotherapy regimen, eg R-CHOP

Chromosome: A small 'package' found in the nucleus (centre) of every cell in the body that contains a set of genes (DNA codes); they occur in pairs, one from the mother and one from the father, and human beings normally possess 46 chromosomes, arranged in 23 pairs

Chronic: A condition, either mild or severe, that lasts for a long time

Classification: The grouping of similar types of cancer together according to how they look under the microscope and after doing specialised tests

Clinical trial: A research study in which people help doctors to find better ways of treating a disease, for example by investigating the effects of a new treatment or aspect of care

CMV: Short for 'cytomegalovirus', a virus that is more likely to cause infections in people whose immune system is weakened by lymphoma or a treatment for lymphoma

Combination chemotherapy: Treatment with more than one chemotherapy drug

Combined modality therapy (CMT): The use of both chemotherapy and radiotherapy in a single course of anti-lymphoma treatment

Complete response: There is no evidence of lymphoma using current tests

CT scan: Short for 'computed tomography', a scan performed in an X-ray department that provides a layered picture of the inside of the body; can be used to detect disease of a tissue or organ

Cure: The treatment of a disease to the point where it has gone and will not come back in the future

Cutaneous: To do with the skin

Cycle A block of chemotherapy that is followed by a rest period to allow the healthy normal cells to recover

Cyto-: To do with cells

Cytogenetics: The study and testing of the chromosomes in cells that are involved in disease; helps to identify different types of lymphoma, reach an accurate diagnosis and aid treatment planning

Cytotoxic drugs: Drugs that are toxic (poisonous) to cells, so are given to destroy or control cancer cells

---

D

Day-care unit A part of the hospital for people who need a specialist procedure but who do not need to stay in hospital overnight

Day patient or outpatient A patient who attends hospital, eg for treatment, but doesn't stay overnight

Diagnosis Naming a condition or disease

Diaphragm The dome-shaped muscle that separates the abdomen from the thoracic (chest) cavity

Disease-free survival The percentage of people who are alive and free of lymphoma after a certain number of years.

Disease progression or progression Continued growth of the lymphoma. This is usually defined as growth of more than a fifth (more than 20%) while you are having treatment

DNA Stands for 'deoxyribonucleic acid', a complex molecule that holds genetic information as a chemical code and which forms part of the chromosome in the nucleus of all the cells of the body

Double-hit lymphoma The lymphoma cells have 2 major lymphoma-related changes in their genes. Usually a type of diffuse large B-cell lymphoma (DLBCL)

E

Early stage Lymphoma that is localised to 1 area or a few areas that are close together, usually stage 1 or 2

Echocardiography The use of sound waves to study the strength of the heart by showing the structure and movement of the heart chambers and heart valves

Efficacy The ability of a drug to produce a beneficial effect

Electrocardiography (ECG) A method of recording the electrical activity of the heart muscle

Endoscopy A procedure in which a flexible optical instrument is passed into an internal organ to assist in diagnosis and treatment (eg in gastroscopy an endoscope is passed through the mouth into the stomach)

Epidemiology The study of how often disease occurs in different groups of people and why (ie the investigation of diseases as they affect whole populations, not individuals)

Epstein–Barr virus (EBV) A commonly occurring herpes virus that causes glandular fever; has been discovered to be associated with some lymphomas, particularly Burkitt lymphoma

Erythrocytes Red blood cells

Erythropoietin A protein hormone produced mainly in the kidneys that stimulates the formation of red blood cells; can be manufactured (as EPO) and is given to some people as a treatment for anaemia, especially if they have kidney failure

Excision biopsy An operation to remove a lump completely; in people with lymphoma this usually means the removal of a whole lymph node

Extranodal disease Lymphoma occurring outside the lymphatic system

---

F

False negative A negative result in a test when that person does have the condition

False positive A positive result in a test when that person does not have the condition

Familial A familial condition runs in a family, showing up in several family members, but it is not associated with a particular identified gene or genetic defect (as in inherited conditions)

Fatigue Feeling of extreme tiredness and lack of energy, a common side effect of cancer and of cancer treatments

Fertility The ability to have children

Fibrosis Thickening and scarring of tissues (eg lymph nodes, the lungs); can happen after an infection, surgery or radiotherapy

Fine-needle aspiration Sometimes shortened to 'FNA', a procedure in which a small amount of fluid and cells is removed from a lump or lymph node using a thin needle; the cells are then examined under a microscope

First-line therapy The first choice of therapy selected to combat an illness when it first appears or if it comes back

Flow cytometry A laboratory technique used to analyse lymphoma cells to help make an accurate diagnosis and plan the best treatment (a kind of immunophenotyping)

Follicle A very small sac or gland; in follicular lymphoma the term relates to the appearance of groups or clusters of lymphoma cells seen under the microscope when a biopsy sample is examined

Fungus A type of organism that can cause disease

G

G-CSF Stands for 'granulocyte colony-stimulating factor', a growth factor that stimulates the bone marrow to make more white blood cells

Gene A stretch of DNA with enough genetic information in it to form a protein

Genetic Caused by the genes

GM-CSF Stands for 'granulocyte and macrophage colony-stimulating factor', a growth factor that stimulates the bone marrow to make more white blood cells and platelets

Grade A way of expressing how fast a lymphoma is growing: low-grade lymphomas are slower growing; high-grade lymphomas are faster growing

Graft-versus-host disease (GvHD) A condition that can occur after an allogeneic stem cell or bone marrow transplant where T cells from the graft (the donated marrow or stem cells) attack some of the normal cells of the host (the person who received the transplant)

Graft-versus-lymphoma effect A similar effect to GvHD but this time a beneficial effect that the donor bone marrow or stem cells have on the host's lymphoma cells, turning on them and killing them; it is not fully understood how this happens

Gray A measure of how much radiation is being absorbed by the body; radiotherapy is 'prescribed' in numbers of Gray (shortened to 'Gy')

Groshong® line A type of central line

Growth factors Naturally occurring complex proteins that control the development of blood cells and their release into the bloodstream; sometimes used during lymphoma treatments to increase the numbers of particular types of white blood cell and the numbers of stem cells circulating in the bloodstream (eg G-CSF, GM-CSF)

H

Haematologist A doctor specialising in diseases of the blood and blood cells, including leukaemias and lymphomas

Haematopoiesis The process of blood cell formation, which takes place in the bone marrow

Haemoglobin An iron-containing protein found in red blood cells that carries oxygen around the body

Helicobacter pylori A bacterium that causes inflammation and ulcers in the stomach and which is associated with a particular lymphoma in the stomach (gastric MALT lymphoma)

Helper T cells T cells that stimulate B cells to make more antibodies as part of the body's immune response

Hickman® line A type of central line

High-dose therapy A treatment regimen in which large doses of anti-cancer treatments are given with the aim of eradicating all the tumour cells; because this will also damage the normal blood-producing cells in the bone marrow it has to be followed by a transplant of either stem cells (a peripheral blood stem cell transplant, PBSCT) or bone marrow cells (a bone marrow transplant, BMT)

Histo- To do with tissue or cells

Histochemistry The study of the chemistry of tissues and cells using specialised stains and chemical reactions

Histology The study of the microscopic appearance and structure of tissues and cells

Histopathologist A doctor who specialises in histopathology

Histopathology The study of the microscopic appearances of diseased tissues

HIV Short for 'human immunodeficiency virus', which is a virus that attacks the immune system and can cause acquired immune deficiency syndrome (AIDS)

Hormone A chemical messenger secreted by a gland and carried by the bloodstream to another part of the body to affect how that part works

Hypothyroidism The condition caused by a lack of thyroid hormone (thyroxine); can occur as a late side effect of radiotherapy to the neck

---

I

Immune system A system in the body that fights infections and causes allergic reactions; consists of white blood cells, the spleen and the lymph nodes

Immunisation The process of making someone immune to something or building up their immune response to it so that they can resist the infection in the future; one way of immunising a person is to introduce an antigen (such as a germ) into the body, which is what happens in vaccination

Immunocompromised Meaning the same as 'immunosuppressed', a condition of reduced ability to resist infection or combat foreign material gaining access to the body; can be caused by a disease or by a treatment

Immunoglobulins Sometimes shortened to 'Ig', the chemical name for antibodies, a group of naturally occurring proteins found in the plasma blood that are involved in our immune system, destroying foreign cells and stimulating other parts of our immune system into action

Immunophenotyping A specialised laboratory technique that is used to study the proteins that are present on the surface of lymphoma cells; helps the doctor to tell the difference between different lymphomas and make an accurate diagnosis

Immunosuppression A condition of reduced immunity caused by a treatment; can allow infections to occur

Immunosuppressive A drug that lowers the body's ability to fight infection

Immunotherapy A treatment that stimulates the body's own immune system to fight a cancer or lymphoma

Indolent Lymphoma that is growing slowly

Infection Bacteria, viruses, parasites or fungi (germs) that don't normally live in the body invade your body and can make you ill. If your immune system is not working well, infections can come from the bacteria that normally live on your body, eg on your skin or in your bowel

Infusion The giving of a fluid other than blood into a vein

Inpatient A patient who stays in hospital overnight.

Intramuscular Into muscle

Intrathecal Into the fluid around the spinal cord

Intravenous Into a vein

Irradiated blood Blood (or platelets) that has been treated with X-rays before transfusion to destroy any white cells; done to prevent transfusion-associated graft-versus-host disease

L

Late effects Health problems due to treatment that develop months or years after treatment has ended

Leukaemia Cancer of the white blood cells

Live vaccine a vaccine that contains a live, weakened version of the microbe (germ) that causes an infection.

Lumbar puncture A technique where some cerebrospinal fluid is removed from the fluid-filled space around the nerves in the spine

Lymph A fluid that circulates in the body's lymph vessels, partially made up of fluid drained from the tissues; it carries salts and large numbers of lymphocytes

Lymphadenopathy Enlargement of lymph nodes

Lymphatic system A system of tubes (lymph vessels), glands (lymph nodes), the thymus and the spleen that helps fight infection and filters waste fluids and cells from the tissues

Lymph nodes Small oval swellings, usually up to 2 cm in length, arranged in groups at various points along the course of the lymphatic drainage system, for example in the neck, armpit and groin; they help the body fight infections and drain away waste fluids from the tissues

Lymph vessels The tubes that carry lymph and connect with the lymph nodes

Lymphocytes Specialised white blood cells concerned in the body's immune system; there are three main types – B cells, T cells and the much less common natural killer (NK) cells

Lymphoid tissue Tissue involved in the production of lymph and lymphocytes; consists of bone marrow and thymus gland (the 'primary' lymphoid organs) and the lymph nodes, spleen, tonsils and some tissue in the gut called Peyer's patches (the 'secondary' lymphoid organs)

Lymphoma A cancer of lymphoid tissue

M

Macrophage A type of white blood cell involved in the immune system that ingests or engulfs foreign organisms and sends out chemical messages to recruit and stimulate other cells of the immune system to strengthen the immune response

Maintenance therapy Treatment to keep lymphoma in remission after successful treatment

Malignant Cancerous, something that grows uncontrollably and can travel to other parts of the body

MALT Stands for 'mucosa-associated lymphoid tissue' and is lymphoid tissue found in lining membranes (known as mucous membranes or mucosa) throughout the body, including the gut, the lungs and the salivary glands

Mediastinum The central part of the chest that contains the heart, the windpipe (trachea), the gullet (oesophagus), important large blood vessels and the lymph nodes around the heart

Medical alert card A card containing information about your condition or treatment. If you are given a medical alert card, you should carry it with you at all times

Metastasis The spread of cancer cells from the site where they originated to other areas of the body

Minimal residual disease (MRD) Tiny amounts of lymphoma remaining after treatment. If you are MRD positive, the remaining disease can grow and cause a relapse. If you are MRD negative, you have a better chance of a long-lasting remission

Monoclonal antibody A protein made to recognise and attach itself to a specific 'marker' antigen protein on the surface of a cell (eg rituximab attaches to an antigen on lymphoma cells called CD20); the immune system is then alerted to destroy the lymphoma cell

MRI Short for 'magnetic resonance imaging', a method of body scanning using a magnetic field to give very detailed images of the inside of the body

Mucosa The tissue that lines most of the body's hollow organs, such as the gut, the air passages and the ducts of glands that open into these hollow organs (such as the salivary glands)

Mucositis Inflammation of the inside (lining) of the mouth

MUGA Short for 'multigated acquisition', this is a type of scan that assesses how well the heart is pumping; sometimes done before starting certain chemotherapy drugs

Myelodysplastic syndromes Sometimes called 'myelodysplasia', a group of diseases in which the normal function of the bone marrow is disrupted and the bone marrow makes defective blood cells instead of healthy ones

Myeloma A cancer of plasma cells (a type of B cell) found in the bone marrow

Myeloproliferative disorders Diseases in which too many of one or more types of blood cell are produced in the bone marrow

---

N

Needle aspiration biopsy Also sometimes known as 'fine-needle aspiration biopsy' or FNAB, a technique in which a thin needle is inserted into a lump (eg a neck lump) to remove some cells to be examined under a microscope

Neuro- To do with nerves or the nervous system

Neuropathy Any disease that affects the nerves (neurones)

Neutropenia Low levels of neutrophils (a kind of white blood cell) in the blood; can result in the body allowing infections to develop

Neutropenic sepsis A severe infection in people with neutropenia due to disease or to lymphoma treatments; sometimes called 'febrile neutropenia' if the temperature is high

Neutrophils Small, short-lived white blood cells that are particularly important in fighting off bacterial infections

NICE Stands for the 'National Institute for Health and Care Excellence', an independent body that gives guidance to the NHS and recommends whether treatments should be funded

---

O

Oncologist A doctor who specialises in the diagnosis and treatment of people with cancer; may be either a medical oncologist who gives drug treatments for cancer or a 'clinical oncologist' (also known as a radiotherapist) who mainly gives radiotherapy

Oral By mouth, eg as a tablet or capsule

Overall survival the percentage of people who are still alive after a certain number of years, with or without lymphoma. Overall survival (OS) is often measured 5 years and 10 years after treatment has ended

---

P

Paediatric To do with children

Palliative Treatment or care designed to help relieve the symptoms of a condition (eg pain) rather than to cure it

Paraprotein An abnormal protein found in the blood or the urine

Parenteral The giving of drugs or nutrients by any other method than by mouth or into the bowel (given instead by intramuscular injection or by intravenous injection or infusion)

Partial response Lymphoma that has decreased by at least a half but there is still lymphoma present.

Pathologist A doctor who studies diseased tissues under a microscope

Performance status A way of expressing how well and active you are; ranges from 0 (fully active) to 4 (bedridden) in the World Health Organisation performance status scale

Peripheral blood stem cell transplant A type of therapy which initially uses high doses of chemotherapy and/or radiotherapy to destroy cancer cells, followed by transplantation of stem cells to replace the damaged bone marrow (this damage being a side effect of the high doses of chemotherapy)

Peripheral neuropathy A condition of nerves outside the brain and spinal cord (the peripheral nervous system), which usually begins in the hands or feet with symptoms of numbness, tingling, burning and/or weakness; can be caused by some lymphomas (eg Waldenström's macroglobulinaemia) and by some anti-cancer drugs

PET Short for 'positron-emission tomography', a scan in which a radioactive tracer chemical is used to detect altered tissue metabolism or cellular activity, for example metabolically active cancer 'hot spots'

PET/CT scan A scan in which PET and CT scans are combined

PICC line Short for 'peripherally inserted central catheter', a central line that is put in at a point further away from the chest than most other central lines (eg in the upper arm)

Placebo An inactive or 'dummy' treatment designed to resemble the drug being tested in a clinical trial. Usually, one group of people taking part in the trial have standard treatment plus the test drug. Another group of people have standard treatment plus the placebo. Used to rule out any psychological effects of taking a treatment

Plasma The fluid part of the blood that the blood cells are suspended in; contains proteins, salts and blood-clotting compounds

Plasma cell A cell that is formed from a B lymphocyte that produces antibodies

Plasmapheresis Sometimes called 'plasma exchange', a procedure where the liquid part of the blood (plasma) is separated from the blood cells using a special apparatus and the cells are returned to the circulation; used to remove protein from the blood of a person with too much of that protein in their blood, eg in Waldenström's macroglobulinaemia

Platelets Found in the blood, these small round bodies (fragments of bigger cells called megakaryocytes) help the blood-clotting process

Portacath A type of central line sometimes used in children that does not come out through the skin but has a needle put into it whenever it needs to be used

Principal treatment centre (PTC) Specialist centre treating children and young people with cancer up to the age of 18

Progenitor cell Sometimes called a 'precursor cell', an immature cell which can develop into a number of different cell types

Prognosis The likely course of an illness for an individual patient, taking many factors into account such as the type of tumour, age and general health

Progression-free interval The time between treatment and the lymphoma starting to increase again. Sometimes called the 'event-free interval'

Progression-free survival The time someone lives without their lymphoma starting to increase again

Protein Matter found in living things with many roles, including helping to control how our cells work and fighting infections

Protocol The plan for a research trial that includes information on the research question being asked by the trial, the eligibility criteria, investigations required and follow-up requirements

R

Radiographer A person who takes radiographs (X-rays) and performs other scans (a diagnostic radiographer) or gives radiotherapy (a therapeutic radiographer)

Radioimmunotherapy A treatment using a monoclonal antibody with a particle of radiation attached to it in order to directly target the lymphoma cell, so giving radiotherapy to the lymphoma cells without affecting the healthy cells nearby

Radiologist A doctor who interprets radiographs (X-rays) and scans; may also perform biopsies using scans to ensure the right bit of tissue is taken to be examined

Radiotherapist A doctor who specialises in treating people using radiotherapy, also known as a 'clinical oncologist'

Radiotherapy Treatment in which powerful, carefully focused beams of radiation (like X-rays) are used to damage and kill lymphoma and other cancer cells; sometimes called 'external beam radiotherapy'

Randomisation A method that ensures that each participant in a clinical trial has the same chance of being put into the different treatment groups

Red blood cells These cells carry oxygen around the body; also known as 'erythrocytes'

Reed–Sternberg cell An abnormal cell with a characteristic appearance under the microscope of 'owl eyes'; if present in a biopsy this would indicate a Hodgkin lymphoma

Refractory Resistant to treatment, meaning that the treatment no longer has an effect on the cancer cells

Regimen A particular course or plan of treatment (eg of drugs, diet, exercise) that is designed to bring about an improvement in health or a condition; usually quite specific and stipulates the dosage and duration if it involves drugs

Relapse The return or recurrence of disease after previous treatment and apparent recovery

Remission A period when there is no evidence of a disease using tests that are currently available (complete remission); a 'partial remission' is when more than half the disease or tumour has melted away after treatment; and a 'good partial remission' is when three-quarters of the tumour has gone

Respiratory Relating to breathing or to the organs of breathing (the lungs and air passages)

Response See also 'complete response' and 'partial response'

S

Scan A test where the inside of the body is looked at from the outside, eg CT scan, ultrasound scan

Sedation Where a relaxing drug is given through a vein to enable a procedure to be done more easily and comfortably

Sedative A relaxing drug given into a vein to make a procedure easier or more comfortable to do

Sepsis Poisoning of the body by the products of infectious organisms such as bacteria and by the chemicals produced by the body as an immune response to the infection

Side effect An unwanted effect of a medical treatment

SMC Stands for the 'Scottish Medicines Consortium', the body that gives guidance to the NHS in Scotland on whether treatments should be funded

Specialist nurse A nurse who has specialised in looking after people with lymphoma who can help you understand more about the disease and its treatment. Your specialist nurse (sometimes called a clinical nurse specialist or CNS) will usually be the first person you should contact about any worries or concerns.

Spleen Part of the immune system, a pear-sized organ lying just under the rib cage on the left-hand side of the body, behind the stomach; involved in fighting infection and acts as a filter of the blood, removing foreign particles and destroying old blood cells

Splenectomy Surgical removal of the spleen

Splenomegaly Enlargement of the spleen

Stable disease Lymphoma that has stayed the same (ie neither gone away nor progressed)

Stage A guide to how many (and which) areas of your body are affected by lymphoma. There are four stages, which are written with Roman numerals as stage I to stage IV

Staging The process of finding out what stage a lymphoma is at; involves examinations and tests

Stem cell harvest The process of collecting stem cells from the blood

Stem cell transplant The process of giving back previously harvested stem cells (an autologous stem cell transplant) or of giving donated stem cells (an allogeneic stem cell transplant)

Stem cells Immature cells which can develop into the different types of mature cells normally found in healthy blood

Steroids Naturally occurring hormones that are involved in many of the body's natural functions; can also be manufactured and given as a treatment

Subcutaneous Under the skin

Surgery Treatment that involves cutting into the body to change or remove something

Symptom Any change in the body or in how it functions that is felt by a person; helps doctors to diagnose diseases

Systemic Affecting the whole body (ie not just local or localised)

T

T cells / T lymphocytes Cells of the immune system that help to protect us from viruses and cancers by attacking them directly; they develop in the thymus gland

Thrombocytopenia A shortage of platelets in the blood; increases the likelihood of bruising and/or bleeding

Thymus A small flat gland situated at the top of the chest, immediately behind the breast bone; the organ where T cells develop

Topical Putting a treatment directly onto the surface of the skin

Total body irradiation Radiotherapy given to the whole body, not just a part of it; usually given to kill off any lymphoma cells left in the body before a stem cell transplant

Transformation Change of one type of tissue or tumour (eg low-grade lymphoma) into another type of tissue or tumour (eg high-grade lymphoma)

Transfusion The giving of blood or blood products (eg red cells, stem cells) into a vein

Transfusion-associated graft-versus-host disease (TA-GvHD) A rare but serious complication of blood or platelet transfusion where white cells in the transfused blood attack the cells of the person receiving the blood; can be prevented by irradiation of blood and platelets

Tumour A swelling or lump of tissue formed from a collection of cells; can be benign or malignant

Tumour flare Sometimes called a 'flare reaction', this is a temporary increase in the lymphoma symptoms after starting treatment and is more common with certain drugs, eg lenalidomide, rituximab (rituximab flare)

Tumour lysis syndrome A rare but serious illness that can occur when dying tumour cells release chemical by-products into the circulation that disturb the metabolism; usually occurs after combination chemotherapy or sometimes after treatment with steroid drugs

Tumour markers A substance whose presence in the blood or urine indicates the possible presence of a tumour in the body

---

V

Vaccination Increasing the body's power to resist an infection by inoculating it with a small dose of the germ or organism that causes that infection (the organism is usually first killed or modified to make it safe); some vaccinations (with live vaccines) are not safe for people with lymphoma

Varicella zoster The virus that causes chickenpox and shingles

Vinca alkaloid Anti-cancer drugs originally derived from a member of the periwinkle (Vinca) plant family; examples are vincristine and vinblastine

Virus A tiny organism that causes disease. Unlike bacteria, viruses are not made up of cells

---

W

White blood cell A cell found in the blood and in many other tissues that helps our bodies to fight infections. There are several different types, including lymphocytes and neutrophils.

X

X-ray A form of radiation that is used to take pictures of the inside of the body and for radiotherapy; also used to mean the picture that is taken (the radiograph)

Introduction

What is lymphoma?

Lymphoma is the fifth most common type of cancer in the UK. It can occur at any age, even in children. It is nearly always treatable; most people live for many years after being diagnosed with lymphoma.

1 Causes of lymphoma

There is no known cause in most cases of lymphoma. This page describes some of the possible factors that could contribute to the development of lymphoma.

2 The lymphatic system

Lymphoma is a cancer of the lymphatic system. The lymphatic system is part of your immune system, which helps protect you from infection. It is spread throughout your body, like blood vessels, and it has many different parts. This page tells you about the different parts of the lymphatic system and what they do.

2.1 What is the lymphatic system and what does it do?

The lymphatic system runs throughout the body, like your blood circulatory system. The lymphatic system carries a fluid called 'lymph' around the body in lymph vessels (tubes). The fluid passes through lymph nodes (glands), which are spread throughout your body.

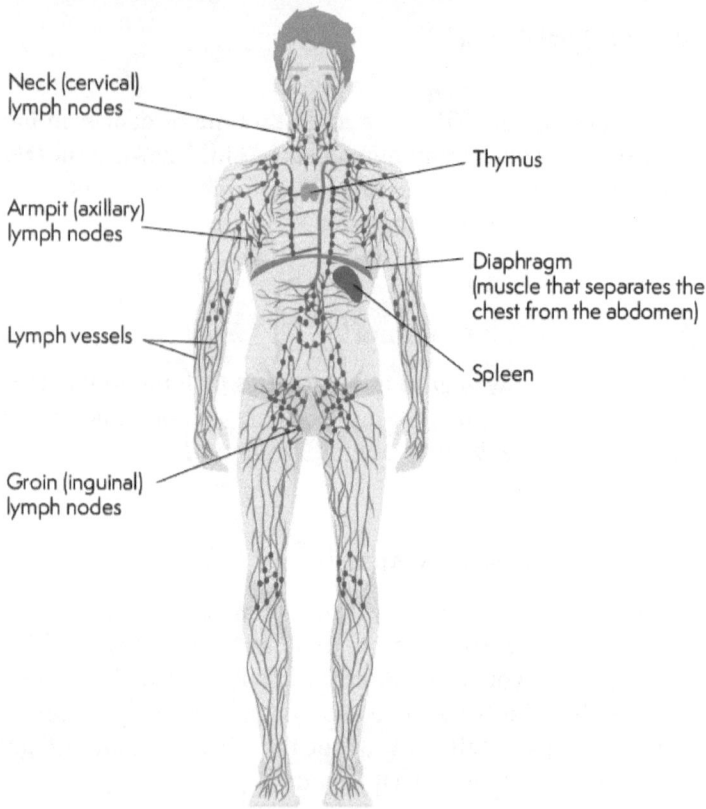

Figure: The lymphatic system (lymph vessels and lymph nodes are shown in green)

The lymphatic system also includes organs and tissues that are places where immune system cells collect. These include the parts of the body that make cells for the immune system:

- the bone marrow
- the thymus.

They also include areas where immune cells collect, ready to fight infection:

- lymph nodes
- the spleen
- the tonsils and adenoids
- mucosa-associated lymphoid tissue.

The lymphatic system defends your body against disease by removing germs (bacteria, viruses and parasites) and toxins (poisons). It also helps to destroy cells that are old, damaged or have become abnormal. It has other important functions too:

- As a drainage system, it removes excess fluid and waste from your tissues and returns it to your bloodstream.
- It helps to absorb fats and fat-soluble vitamins from your digestive system and to transport them to your bloodstream.

The whole of the lymphatic system helps to protect us against infection. Any part of it can be affected by lymphoma.

- Lymph
- Lymph is a clear fluid that flows around the body in the lymphatic system. It is formed from plasma. Plasma is carried around your body in your blood vessels. It leaks out of the blood vessels and bathes your tissues and supplies the

cells of your body with nutrients. Most of this plasma then drains back into the blood vessels. A small amount is left behind, together with:

- waste products from the cells
- fat that is broken down in the bowel and needs to be carried to larger blood vessels
- things that have got into the body and might be harmful, such as germs and toxins
- damaged or abnormal cells, including cancer cells.
- This all drains into tiny lymph vessels. Lymph vessels in the small intestine also absorb fats and fat-soluble vitamins.
- When it is in lymph vessels, the fluid is known as 'lymph'.
- The lymph flows from the tiny lymph vessels into larger lymph vessels, heading towards one of two lymphatic ducts. The lymph filters through lymph nodes as it flows around your body. The lymph nodes contain lots of lymphocytes (white blood cells that fight infection). Anything that doesn't belong in your body, and any damaged and abnormal cells are removed in the lymph nodes. Lymph leaving the lymph nodes also carries lymphocytes. These lymphocytes can fight infections elsewhere in the body if needed.
- When the lymph reaches the lymphatic ducts, it goes into your bloodstream, draining into the large veins close to your heart. This removes excess fluid from around your body, helping to maintain your blood pressure and to avoid swelling.
- Unlike blood, lymph is not pumped around your body by the heart. Instead, it is pushed along when your lymph vessels are squeezed by your muscles, and by gravity if the

vessel is above the heart. It is a one-way system: valves stop any lymph flowing backwards.

Lymph nodes

- Lymph nodes are small, bean-shaped structures. They are usually around 1cm long, although this can vary depending on where they are in the body. There are thousands of them throughout the body.

Lymph nodes filter the lymph from nearby parts of the body.

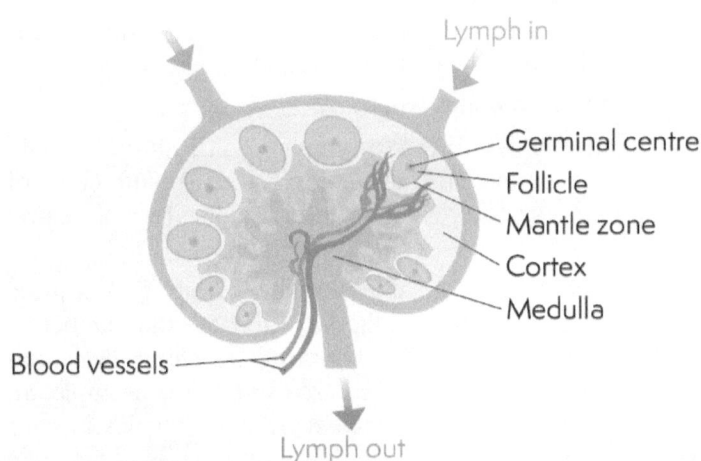

-

Structure of a lymph node

- Where are lymph nodes found?
- There are lymph nodes at various points along the lymph vessels. They are often grouped together. There are groups of lymph nodes all around your body, except your brain and spinal cord. For example, groups of lymph nodes are found in the:

- neck (cervical nodes)
- armpits (axillary nodes)
- groin (inguinal nodes)
- centre of the chest between the lungs (mediastinal nodes)
- abdomen, which is your tummy area.
- Some lymph nodes can be felt from the outside if they swell up, for example those in the neck, armpit or groin. If these lymph nodes swell, you might be able to feel a lump in that area. This often happens if you have an infection and is not usually a sign of something serious. There are also lots of lymph nodes deep within your body. These lymph nodes can't be felt from the outside but can be seen on scans.
- **How do lymph nodes work?**
- The lymph nodes filter the lymph passing through them. They trap germs (for example, bacteria) and cells of the immune system that give information about a nearby infection.
- If there are signs of an infection, your body makes more lymphocytes to help fight the infection. As the number of lymphocytes builds up, the lymph nodes along the lymph vessels that drain the infected area swell. For example, an infection in the throat can cause the lymph nodes in your neck to swell.
- When the infection has been destroyed, most of the immune system cells that were made in response to the infection die off. The lymph nodes normally return to their usual size in a couple of weeks. Most swollen lymph nodes are due to infections. If lymphoma cells collect in the lymph nodes, the swelling does not go down.

- Bone marrow
- Bone marrow is the spongy material at the centre of many of your bones. It makes all the new blood cells you need, including red blood cells, platelets and the different white blood cells.

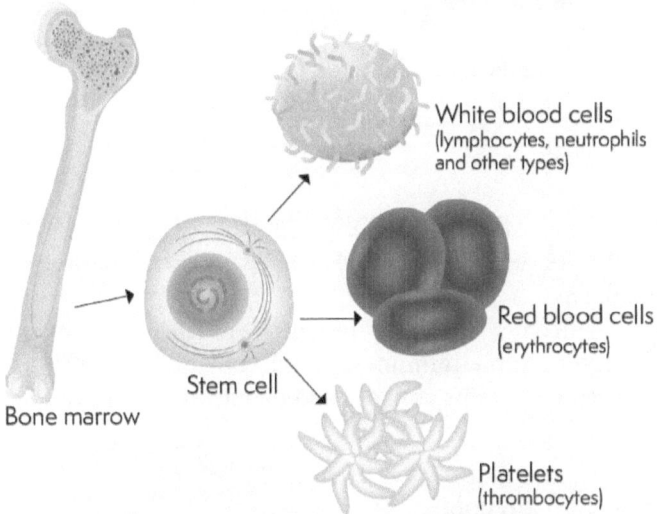

Bone marrow and the blood cells it produces

- White blood cells are involved in the fight against infection. Lymphocytes are white blood cells that are part of the lymphatic system. They are the cells that become abnormal in lymphoma.
- There are two types of lymphocytes: B lymphocytes (B cells) and T lymphocytes (T cells). Both are made in the bone marrow, then live throughout the lymphatic system.

Thymus

- The thymus is a small, butterfly-shaped gland in your chest. It sits behind your breastbone, just above your heart. It grows until puberty and then gradually shrinks in adults. T cells develop into fully working T cells in the thymus. When fully developed, they enter the bloodstream and lymphatic system.
- As adults, T cells are maintained through division of mature T cells outside of the central lymphoid organs.

Spleen

- The spleen is a pear-sized organ that lies just under your rib cage on the left-hand side of your body, behind your stomach.
- The spleen filters blood, much like lymph nodes filter lymph. Immune system cells that live in your spleen remove germs, and old and damaged cells from your blood.

Tonsils and adenoids

- Your tonsils and adenoids are at the back of your throat and nose. They contain lots of immune system cells that help protect your body against infections that enter through the mouth and nose.

Mucosa-associated lymphoid tissue

- Mucosal tissue is the soft, moist, protective tissue that lines many parts of your body, for example your mouth, gut, breathing passages and other internal organs.
- Mucosa-associated lymphoid tissue (MALT) is an area in the mucosa where lymphocytes and other immune system cells collect together. MALT can be found in the wall of the bowel (where it is known as 'Peyer's patches') and in other organs, such as the lungs, eyes, nose and the thyroid gland.
- MALT helps protect the body from infections and toxins entering through a part of the body lined by mucosa. The immune cells in MALT fight the infection or remove any toxins from your body.
- MALT can form when healthy lymphocytes collect in tissue outside lymph nodes in response to an infection or inflammation (a reaction to injury, irritation or infection). This is a normal process. However, MALT lymphomas can develop when abnormal lymphocytes collect in this lymphoid tissue.

The lymphatic system and lymphoma

Lymphocytes are part of the lymphatic system and are spread throughout the body. When lymphocytes become abnormal, lymphoma can develop. Lymphoma can therefore develop in almost any part of the body. It is also easy for lymphoma to spread throughout the body in the lymphatic system. Unlike other cancers, most people with lymphoma have it in more than one place when they are diagnosed. Lymphoma that is in lots of places in the body can be successfully treated and often cured.

3 The immune system

Lymphocytes, the cancerous cells in lymphoma, are a type of immune system cell. This page tells you about how the immune system works.

3.1 What is the immune system?

Your immune system protects your body against infection and disease. It recognises the cells that belong to your body and tries to get rid of anything that shouldn't be there in case it causes you harm. This includes germs (bacteria, viruses and parasites) and toxins (poisons). Your immune system also helps to destroy cells that are old, damaged or have become abnormal.

There are different parts of your immune system, which work in different ways. There are also different types of immunity.

You have 'innate immunity', which you are born with. This includes:

- physical barriers that prevent organisms getting into your body
- phagocytes (types of immune cell), which can fight lots of different types of infection and disease.

You also develop 'acquired immunity' throughout your life as you get exposed to infections. This type of immunity is specific to those infections and prevents you getting the same infections again. Vaccinations expose you to a small dose or inactivated form of the infection so that your immune system can recognise it in future. Lymphocytes (a type of white blood cell or immune cell) are important for acquired immunity. They 'remember' infections you have had before so your body can produce lots of immune system cells very quickly if you are exposed to the same infection again. Lymphocytes are also the immune cells that become abnormal in lymphoma.

3.2 Physical barriers

Physical barriers are the first-line of protection against infection. They include your:

- skin
- mucosa (sometimes called mucous membranes) – the soft, moist lining in certain areas of the body, such as your mouth, nose, gut, and breathing passages.

Your skin prevents any germs getting into your body and also produces oils that can help kill them.

Fluids, such as tears and saliva, wash away germs on the mucosa. Parts of the mucosa also produce sticky mucus, for example, phlegm in your breathing passages. The mucus can trap germs. Proteins and immune cells in the mucus attack and destroy these germs.

Your stomach acid helps to destroy any germs that you swallow.

Immune cells

If a germ gets past your body's physical barriers, you have lots of immune cells to fight infection. There are different types of immune cells. Most of these are types of white blood cell.

Immune cells can be divided into phagocytes and lymphocytes.

3.2.1 Phagocytes

Phagocytes can 'eat' or destroy germs and any of your own cells that are no longer useful to your body. There are several different types, including:

- **Macrophages**, which develop from white blood cells called 'monocytes'. They 'eat' germs and dead, old or abnormal cells. Macrophages can deal with only small numbers of cells. They use chemical messages to signal for help from other immune cells.
- **Neutrophils**, which are found in your bone marrow and bloodstream but move into tissues if there is an infection. Like macrophages, they kill and destroy germs, particularly fungi and bacteria, and send out more signals to bring other immune cells to the area.

3.2.2 Lymphocytes and antibodies

Lymphocytes are important in giving you immunity (a rapid immune response) to an infection when you have already had that infection in the past. Antibodies are proteins made by lymphocytes to fight infection.

B lymphocytes (B cells)

B cells are made in the bone marrow but live mainly in lymph nodes (glands) and other lymphatic tissues, such as the spleen.

After they've come into contact with an infection, B cells can turn into 'plasma cells' which despite their name, are nothing to do with the liquid part of blood (which is called 'plasma'). Plasma cells produce a huge range of antibodies (proteins that are also known as immunoglobulins).

Antibodies fight infection by sticking to proteins on the surface of invading organisms. These proteins are known as 'antigens'. Each B cell can react to only one type of antigen. If a B cell is triggered by contact with its specific antigen, it quickly makes copies of itself. These copies can turn into plasma cells and produce large amounts of antibody.

Antibodies fight infection by:

- directly stopping the germ getting into our cells
- telling other immune cells (for example, macrophages and neutrophils) that the cell should be destroyed
- switching on proteins called 'complement' to destroy the cells.

They can also stick to toxins (poisons) and stop them doing any harm.

Once the infection has gone, most of the B cells and plasma cells that have been produced in response to the infection die. A few plasma cells remain in the bone marrow for much longer, making antibodies to protect against future infection. A few B cells continue to live in lymph nodes. These can respond again more quickly to the same infection if needed – they are known as 'memory B cells'.

T lymphocytes (T cells)

T cells are made in the bone marrow but develop fully in the thymus, before moving to live in lymph nodes.

Your own cells 'show' antigens to T cells. For example:

- some immune system cells can break down a germ and 'show' antigens to a T cell
- if your own cells are infected, for example with a virus, the T cell can recognise the foreign proteins

- if your own cells become abnormal, they are recognised as different by T cells.

Each T cell can recognise just one type of antigen. If it comes into contact with that antigen, it makes copies of itself. The new cells then become various special types of T cell that work in different ways:

- **Cytotoxic T cells** kill the germ, particularly viruses and tuberculosis (TB) bacteria. They also look out for any of your own cells that might be 'going wrong' (such as becoming a cancer cell) and kill them too.
- **Helper T cells** support the fight against infection by telling B cells to make more antibodies and by 'switching on' more macrophages and neutrophils.
- **Memory T cells** are left behind once the infection has gone – only a few of them are needed. They allow the immune system to respond quickly if the same infection starts again.

NK cells (natural killer cells) are like T cells, except that they do not develop in the thymus. They don't need to be activated by an antigen but recognise signals from your own cells that tell the NK cells not to kill them. They kill cells that have been infected by a virus or are turning into cancer.

3.2.3 Immune cells and proteins that help lymphocytes

Dendritic cells help direct the work of both B cells and T cells. They show antigens from the infection to these cells in a way that tells them to start attacking that infection. They also help the immune system remember infections so it can act quickly when needed again.

Histiocytes are immune cells that stay in one place in the tissues rather than circulating around the body. They can also tell the lymphocytes that an infection is present.

Complement is the name of a group of proteins that are made in the liver and found in the bloodstream. The proteins are switched on by contact with germs and by antibodies. Once switched on, the complement proteins change so that they join together and stick to the germ. They then either punch holes in the germ to burst it or signal to macrophages to 'eat' it.

3.3 What can go wrong with the immune system?

The immune system does not always work perfectly. It might over-react, causing allergies and autoimmune conditions. It might not work as well as it should, causing immunodeficiency. Problems with your immune system can also contribute to the development of lymphoma. Sometimes the immune system does not recognise abnormal cells, which can allow cancer to develop.

3.3.1 The immune system and cancer

As well as protecting you from invading viruses, fungi and bacteria, your immune system should also protect you from your own cells if they go wrong. You might hear this called 'cancer surveillance'.

When a cancer (such as a lymphoma) develops, it means that the immune system, for some reason, has not detected the cancerous cells or has not been able to get rid of them. This does not always mean that the immune system was weak. Often it happens because the cancerous cells looked, on the surface, very like a normal cell. They didn't stand out and therefore weren't detected by the immune system and were able to start growing. Cancer cells also develop ways to prevent the immune system attacking them. For example, some cancer cells make special proteins on their surface that tell T cells not to attack them.

3.4 What is cancer?

Your body is made up of many different types of cell, e.g. skin, bone and blood cells, among others. Your cells grow and divide to form new cells. These new cells replace cells that have grown old or become damaged and died. Cell division and cell death are normal processes that occur in your body. These processes are controlled by chemical signals.

4 Lymphoma and the immune system

Ways in which the immune system is affected by lymphoma

4.1 How does lymphoma affect the immune system?

Lymphomas are due to cancerous lymphocytes (either B cells or T cells). As lymphocytes are part of the immune system, some parts of the immune system may not work as well as normal in people who have lymphoma. Even if they are not cancerous, other cells of your immune system might not work as well as usual if you have lymphoma, because the different parts of the immune system work together.

- If you have T-cell lymphoma, you might not have enough normal T cells to fight infection. A shortage of T cells increases your risk of developing viral infections (for example, shingles and viruses that cause cold sores) and tuberculosis (TB).

- If you have B-cell lymphoma, you might not have enough normal B cells to fight infection. A shortage of B cells increases your risk of bacterial infections (for example, pneumonia and urinary tract infections).
- Lymphoma in the bone marrow can take up the space needed for normal blood cells to develop, including other types of white blood cell that fight infection, such as neutrophils.

Cancer cells, including lymphoma cells, also use up your body's energy. This can affect your immune system's ability to work well and can result in weight loss and loss of muscle mass.

4.2 How does treatment for lymphoma affect the immune system?

Lots of cancer treatments affect the immune system. Treatments for lymphoma aim to kill the cancerous lymphocytes. However, these treatments also kill some of your body's healthy cells, including immune cells. Different types and intensities of treatment affect your body differently.

4.2.1 Effects of treatment on your immune system

Chemotherapy causes damage to bone marrow, which is where your blood cells are made. Your body might not be able to make as many blood cells as usual, reducing your blood counts. Many people treated with chemotherapy develop neutropenia (a shortage of neutrophils). Neutropenia increases your risk of infection, particularly infections due to bacteria. Certain drugs, such as fludarabine, can also lower your number of lymphocytes. This can increase the risk of infection.

Steroids can increase your risk of infections, particularly those caused by viruses (such as those that cause cold sores and chickenpox) and fungi (such as thrush).

Stem cell transplants can have a greater effect on the immune system than most other treatments. This is because they involve high doses of chemotherapy (and sometimes radiotherapy too) that kill cancer cells but also kill the cells in the bone marrow that make immune cells. If you have a stem cell transplant, you also have other treatments (called anti-infection 'prophylaxis') to protect your body from infection until your immune system has recovered.

A splenectomy is an operation to remove the spleen. A few people with lymphoma have a splenectomy. Having no spleen can increase your risk of infection with certain bacteria. If you have a splenectomy, you usually have antibiotics and vaccinations to reduce the risk of infections.

4.2.2 Other ways treatment can affect your immune system

Anything that damages the physical barriers of your immune system can increase your risk of infection. Needles pass through the skin barrier. They are needed to put treatments into your bloodstream and for blood to be taken for blood tests. The tiny holes the needles make in your skin can give germs a way to get into your bloodstream. Lines that stay in place for a while, such as central lines and drips, give more opportunities for infection to develop. Surgery, including biopsies (where a sample of tissue is removed) also create a break in your skin that can allow germs into your body. Your medical team take great care to avoid introducing infections when performing any procedures. They also regularly check lines and wounds and keep them clean. Tell your medical team if you notice any signs of infection, such as redness, swelling or pain at the affected area.

Some people get dry mucous membranes or a sore mouth during treatment for lymphoma. These problems are most common with radiotherapy to the head and neck and some chemotherapy, particularly at high doses. The mucous membranes work as a physical barrier to protect you from infection. If they are dry and sore, they are not working well, which gives organisms more opportunity to enter your body. If you have these problems, there are things you can do to soothe any discomfort and to help prevent infection. Your medical team might be able to give you treatments to reduce your risk of infection.

Your skin can also be affected by the lymphoma itself or as a side effect of treatments for lymphoma. You might develop dry, sore or itchy skin. It is important that you follow any advice from your medical team to avoid introducing infections through broken skin.

4.3 The immune system after treatment

Your immune system should recover over time after your treatment for lymphoma. Most people who have recovered after standard treatment for lymphoma and are in remission are not at increased risk of infection. Some treatments can have longer-term or permanent effects on the immune system, for example:

- Splenectomy - the increased risk of infection lowers over time but never goes away completely. Be vigilant for signs of infection and follow any advice from your medical team.
- Stem cell transplants – it takes many months to recover from a stem cell transplant. If you had an allogeneic stem cell transplant (where you were given donor stem cells), you will need immunosuppressive drugs (drugs that dampen your immune system) after your transplant to stop your new donor immune system from attacking your own cells. Many healthy cells, including immune cells, are also killed by the treatment. This means your immune system is very low after a transplant and it can take more than a year to recover. Most people need to have their childhood vaccinations again after having an allogeneic stem cell transplant.
- Certain chemotherapy drugs that affect lymphocytes, for example fludarabine (often used to treat chronic lymphocytic leukaemia) - problems with immunity can persist for a year or two after treatment. The increased risk of infection generally decreases over time.

It is only natural to feel concerned if you have symptoms of infection or swollen lymph nodes after you have been treated for lymphoma. Everybody gets infections from time to time. If you have neutropenia or are having treatment for lymphoma, infections can be more serious and you should seek medical advice immediately if you suspect you have an infection. If you are in remission and have a normal neutrophil count, you should only worry if your lymph nodes do not shrink back down after the infection has gone.

Always contact your medical team if you are worried about infection or any new or worsening symptoms.

4.4 Using the immune system to treat lymphoma

Some lymphoma treatments use the immune system to help treat the lymphoma. These include:

- Antibody therapy, which uses man-made antibodies to mark out lymphoma cells and tell your immune system to kill them. For example, rituximab is an antibody used to treat many types of lymphoma. Antibody therapy is often used in combination with chemotherapy. This might be known as 'chemo immunotherapy'.
- Allogeneic stem cell transplants, which give you a new immune system from a donor. The new immune system can recognise and attack lymphoma cells. This is known as the 'graft-versus-lymphoma' effect.
- Targeted drugs that can change the way your immune system works or help your immune system to recognise lymphoma cells, for example, immunomodulatory like lenalidomide and checkpoint inhibitors like nivolumab.
- CAR-T cell therapy, where your own T cells are genetically modified (changed) in a laboratory to recognise lymphoma cells before being given back to you.

If a lymphoma develops in someone who is taking immunosuppressive drugs, reducing or stopping those drugs may allow the immune system to get rid of the lymphoma.

Newer drugs and CAR-T cell therapy show promise for treating lymphoma but clinical trials continue to be done to find out more about these treatments and how best to use them.

Symptoms of lymphoma

The most common symptoms of lymphoma, why they happen, and what to do if you have them. Coping with symptoms when diagnosed with lymphoma.

- Common symptoms of lymphoma
- B symptoms
- Swollen lymph nodes
- Fatigue
- Unexplained weight loss
- Night sweats
- Itching
- Fever
- Difficulty getting over infections
- Chest symptoms
- Abdominal (tummy) symptoms
- Pain
- Skin symptoms
- Brain and nerve symptoms
- Swelling in the arms or legs
- Anaemia (low red blood cells)

- There are over 60 types of lymphoma, broadly divided into Hodgkin lymphoma and non-Hodgkin lymphoma. These lymphomas can start almost anywhere in the body and can have many different symptoms. The exact symptoms they cause depend on the type of lymphoma and where it is in the body.

➢ Most of the symptoms of lymphoma can also be symptoms of many other illnesses. These are often mild illnesses such as infections but they can sometimes be more serious conditions.

➢ Because the symptoms of lymphoma are very general, it can sometimes be difficult to diagnose.

➢ The most common symptoms of lymphoma are:

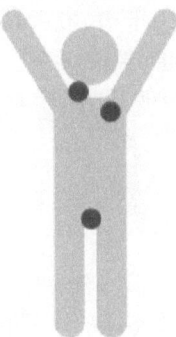

➢ Swollen lymph nodes

➢ The most common sign of lymphoma is a lump or lumps, usually in the neck, armpit or groin. They are usually painless. These lumps are swollen lymph nodes. Lots of things that aren't lymphoma can cause lumps – and not all lymphomas cause obvious lumps.

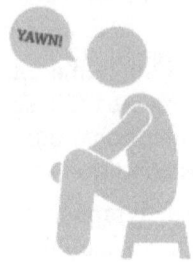

- Fatigue
- Fatigue means being exhausted for no obvious reason or feeling washed out after doing very little. It is not the same as normal tiredness; fatigue is overwhelming and doesn't usually feel better after sleep or rest. Fatigue can be caused by many different things. Lymphoma is just one of them.

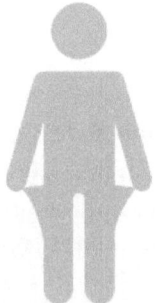

- Unexplained weight loss
- Unexplained weight loss means losing a lot of weight quite quickly when you're not trying to. It can be a symptom of lymphoma – but it can be caused by other things, too.

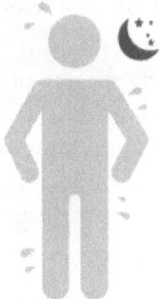

- Sweats
- Lymphoma can cause night sweats that make your nightclothes and bed sheets soaking wet. The night sweats are often described as 'drenching'. They can happen with any type of lymphoma and can also happen during the day. Night sweats can also have causes other than lymphoma.

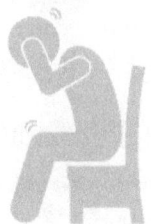

- Itching
- Itching ('pruritus') without a rash can be a symptom of lymphoma but it can have many other causes. It can be very troublesome, particularly in hot weather.

- Lymphoma affects everybody differently. For example:
- You might have lots of symptoms, only a few symptoms, or no symptoms at all. (Sometimes lymphoma is discovered during tests for something else.)
- You might have symptoms in one area (local symptoms) or symptoms that affect your whole body (systemic symptoms).
- You might feel well or you might become very unwell quickly.
- Local symptoms and systemic symptoms
- Some symptoms of lymphoma affect the area in and around the lymphoma itself. These are called 'local symptoms'. The most common local symptom is a swollen lymph node or nodes. Other local symptoms are caused by swollen nodes pressing on nearby tissues. The symptoms you experience depend on where the swollen lymph nodes are. You might have:
- chest symptoms, such as cough or breathlessness
- abdominal (tummy) symptoms, such as a sense of fullness
- skin symptoms, such as a rash or itching
- pain (although this is uncommon)
- brain and nerve symptoms (again, these are uncommon), such as fits (seizures), dizziness or weakness in an arm or leg

- ➢ swelling in your arms or legs
- ➢ anaemia (low numbers of red blood cells), which can make you feel tired.
- ➢ Some symptoms of lymphoma affect your whole body. These are called 'systemic symptoms'. They are caused by the chemicals produced by the lymphoma itself and your body's reaction to the lymphoma. Systemic symptoms include:
- ➢ weight loss
- ➢ fever
- ➢ night sweats
- ➢ fatigue
- ➢ itching
- ➢ frequent infections.
- ➢ Around 1 in 4 people with Hodgkin lymphoma and 1 in 3 people with high-grade non-Hodgkin lymphoma may have systemic symptoms. Systemic symptoms are less common in people with low-grade non-Hodgkin lymphoma.
- ➢ What should I do if I have symptoms of lymphoma?
- ➢ Most of the symptoms of lymphoma can occur in other, more common illnesses as well. Having one or more of these symptoms doesn't necessarily mean you have lymphoma.
- ➢ **If you think you might have lymphoma, or you are worried about any aspect of your health, visit your doctor.**
- ➢ You can also find helpful information and advice about your health on NHS Choices or Patient. Info.

➢ If you have a diagnosis of lymphoma and you're finding it difficult to manage your symptoms, we have some general guidance for coping with some of the common symptoms of lymphoma. Speak to your doctor for advice about managing your individual symptoms.

B symptoms
➢ You may hear the term 'B symptoms', especially when your lymphoma is being staged. Staging is the process of working out how many different parts of your body are affected by lymphoma. The following symptoms are referred to as B symptoms:
➢ unexplained weight loss
➢ night sweats
➢ fever.
➢ Doctors will take into account whether you have any B symptoms when they plan your treatment

---

➢ Swollen lymph nodes
➢ Lymph nodes help to fight infection. They can become swollen for lots of reasons, even when they're working as they should.
➢ A swollen lymph node or nodes is the most common symptom of lymphoma – but lymphoma is **not** the most common cause of swollen lymph nodes. Most people who have swollen lymph nodes do not have lymphoma. More common causes of swollen lymph nodes include:

- infections, such as coughs, colds, ear and throat infections
- illnesses that affect the immune system, such as rheumatoid arthritis
- severe skin diseases such as eczema or psoriasis
- some medicines.
- Swollen lymph nodes caused by infections are usually sensitive or painful to the touch. The swelling normally goes down within 2 or 3 weeks

---

- Swollen lymph nodes caused by lymphoma:
- are most commonly found in the neck, armpit or groin
- are usually smooth and round
- tend to be mobile (they move out of the way when you press on them)
- have a 'rubbery' texture
- are usually painless – although they can sometimes ache or cause pain in nearby areas (for example, if they're pressing on a nerve)
- rarely, can become painful a few minutes after drinking alcohol (this affects up to 5 in 100 people with Hodgkin lymphoma and is probably due to blood vessels in the lymph node widening in response to alcohol).

- **Having swollen lymph nodes does not necessarily mean you have lymphoma. If you notice a lump that doesn't go away within 2 to 3**

weeks, or you find that a lump is getting bigger, see your doctor.

- Lymph nodes in the neck, armpit or groin are close to the surface of the skin and are easy to see and feel. Others, such as those deep inside the abdomen (stomach) or the chest, can't be felt from the outside. If these swell, they might cause pain if they press on internal tissues, or they might only be found on a scan.
- Around 2 in 3 people with lymphoma have swollen lymph nodes that they can feel. It might be the only sign that anything is wrong.
- You might have swollen lymph nodes:
- **in just one area of your body**, which can happen with any type of lymphoma
- **spread throughout your body** (known as 'generalised lymphadenopathy'), which is more common in non-Hodgkin lymphoma than Hodgkin lymphoma.
- Swollen lymph nodes in lymphoma are caused by a build-up of cancerous cells in the lymph nodes. Sometimes the disease is active, making lots of cancerous cells, while at other times it quietens down and some of the cells die. This means the swollen lymph nodes can sometimes grow and shrink, especially in people with low-grade non-Hodgkin lymphoma.

- Fatigue
- Fatigue is overwhelming physical, emotional or mental exhaustion for no obvious reason. It isn't relieved by sleep or rest. People describe it as feeling drained of energy, or being so tired you can't do your normal activities. Sometimes even simple daily tasks, such as getting dressed, can feel too much.
- Many conditions can make you feel fatigued, including anaemia (low red blood cell count), underactive thyroid, depression and anxiety, chronic fatigue syndrome and glandular fever. If you feel fatigued, it does not necessarily mean that you have lymphoma.
- Exactly why lymphoma causes fatigue is not known. It is likely that there are several reasons for it.
- **If you are experiencing fatigue, speak to your doctor.** We also have some suggestions that may help you cope with fatigue.

- Unexplained weight loss
- 'Unexplained' weight loss means losing weight over a short period of time without trying to. The NHS advises that you see your GP if you lose more than 5% of your normal body weight over 6 to 12 months. For an average person, this means losing around half a stone (7lbs) or more. People with lymphoma might lose more than this: over 10% of their body weight within 6 months. For example, a

person who usually weighs 11 stone (70kg) might lose 15lbs (7kg) or more.

➢ Weight loss can happen in people with lymphoma because cancerous cells use up your energy resources. In addition, your body uses energy trying to get rid of the cancerous cells. Weight loss is more common with lymphomas that grow very quickly and put a sudden demand on your body.

➢ As with many other symptoms, weight loss can happen for a lot of other reasons, such as stress, depression, diseases of the digestive tract, or overactive thyroid. Lymphoma is just one of the possible causes of unexplained weight loss.

➢ **Contact your doctor if you lose more than 5% of your body weight over 6 to 12 months without trying to.**

➢ Night sweats
➢ If you have night sweats, it does not necessarily mean you have lymphoma. Night sweats can also be caused by other conditions, such as a viral infection, anxiety, menopause or some medicines.

➢ Doctors don't know exactly why lymphoma causes night sweats. One possible reason is that they are your body's natural reaction to your temperature rising above a normal level (fever). Night sweats may also be a response to some of the chemicals produced by the lymphoma cells.

➢ Lymphoma can cause night sweats that are severe enough to make your nightclothes and bed linen soaking wet. They are often described as 'drenching'. They can happen with any type of lymphoma. Although they are usually called night sweats, they can also sometimes happen during the day.

➢ There are things you can do that might help you to cope with night sweats, but do also speak to your medical team for advice.

➢ **Contact your doctor if you have night sweats that regularly wake you up or if you also have other symptoms, such as fever or unexplained weight loss.**

➢ Itching
➢ Itching (also known as 'pruritus') can be caused by many different conditions, including allergies, skin conditions such as eczema, skin infections or menopause. It is not usually serious. Although itching is common in people with lymphoma, having itchy skin does not necessarily mean you have lymphoma.
➢ Itching affects around 1 in 3 people with Hodgkin lymphoma and 1 in 10 people with non-Hodgkin lymphoma. It can affect:
➢ areas of skin near lymph nodes that are affected by lymphoma
➢ patches of skin lymphoma
➢ the lower legs
➢ the whole body.

- Itching in lymphoma is thought to be due to chemicals released by your immune system, as part of its reaction against the lymphoma cells. These chemicals irritate the nerves in your skin and make it itch.
- Itching due to lymphoma can be severe. It may also cause a burning sensation. It is not usually associated with an obvious rash unless you have skin lymphoma.
- Itching can be very difficult to tolerate, especially in hot weather. It is usually worse at night in bed. If you have a diagnosis of lymphoma and you are struggling to cope with itching, there are some things you could try that might help. Also speak to your medical team for advice.
- **Contact your doctor if you have itching that affects your whole body or lasts for more than 2 weeks.**

- Fever
- Fever is a rise in your body temperature above the normal level. It is almost always caused by an infection, but there are a few other much less common causes, including lymphoma.
- Lymphoma causes fevers because the lymphoma cells produce chemicals that raise your body temperature. Lymphoma usually causes mild fevers a body temperature over 38°C or 100.4°F. These are described as 'low-grade' fevers. They usually come and go.

> **Contact your doctor if you have a fever without an obvious infection that lasts for 2 weeks or more.**

> Difficulty getting over infections
> Having lymphoma can mean that your immune system doesn't work as well as it should.
> Normally, white blood cells fight infections. If you have lymphoma, cancerous white blood cells (that make up the lymphoma) are produced instead of the healthy, 'good' white blood cells. This can make you pick up infections more easily. The infections could be more severe or last for longer than they would normally.
> Infections often cause a high temperature and make you feel hot and shivery. Other symptoms depend on where in your body you have the infection – for example, you might have an earache, a cough, a sore throat, pain when you have a wee, or sickness and diarrhoea.
> **See your doctor if you are worried that you're not getting better after a minor infection.**

> Chest symptoms
> Any type of lymphoma can cause swollen lymph nodes in the chest but they are especially common in Hodgkin lymphoma and some types of high-grade non-Hodgkin lymphoma (where the cells appear to be dividing quickly). Around 1 in 2

people with Hodgkin lymphoma have swollen lymph nodes in their chest.

➢ Swollen lymph nodes in the chest can press on your airways, lungs, or blood vessels. They can also make fluid collect around your lungs. This can cause:

➢ a dry cough
➢ shortness of breath
➢ noisy breathing
➢ pain behind the breastbone
➢ a feeling of pressure in the chest.
➢ These symptoms may be worse when you lie down.
➢ It is important to remember that all these symptoms can happen with many other illnesses, especially lung diseases. Having these symptoms doesn't necessarily mean you have lymphoma.
➢ **Visit your doctor if you have had a cough lasting more than 3 weeks or shortness of breath lasting more than 4 weeks.**

➢ Abdominal (tummy) symptoms
➢ Lymphoma can develop in lymph nodes in the abdomen (tummy) or lymphatic tissue in your liver or spleen. It can also develop outside your lymphatic system ('extranodal' lymphoma). The gut is the most common place for extranodal lymphoma to develop.
➢ Symptoms of lymphoma in the tummy depend on what part of the tummy is involved. For example:

- If your spleen is very swollen, you might have pain behind your ribs on the left side, or you might feel bloated or full after eating only small amounts of food. You or your doctor might be able to feel the swollen spleen as a lump in the top left hand side of your tummy.
- If you have lymphoma affecting your liver, your tummy might become swollen, the whites of your eyes and your skin might develop a yellow tinge (jaundice), or you might notice a build-up of fluid in your abdomen. This can make you feel bloated.
- Lymphoma in the stomach can cause inflammation of the stomach lining (gastritis), which may cause pain, nausea (feeling sick) and vomiting.
- Lymphoma in the bowel can cause abdominal pain, diarrhoea or constipation.
- **See your doctor if you have blood in your faeces, diarrhoea for more than 7 days, green or yellow vomit, vomiting lasting more than 2 days, or if you are dehydrated and you are unable to keep liquids down.**
- **See your doctor urgently if your skin or the whites of your eyes look yellow.**

Pain
- Swollen lymph nodes themselves are not usually painful but lymphoma can press on the tissues around the nodes and cause pain. Where you feel the pain depends on where the lymphoma is.

> Lymphoma in the bone itself is rare but when it does happen, it can cause pain in the affected bone. It is more common to have lymphoma in the bone marrow (the spongy part in the middle of some of our larger bones), but this doesn't usually cause pain.

Suspect then see a doctor.

> Skin symptoms
> If you have skin lymphoma, you might get symptoms on your skin such as:
> flat red patches
> raised plaques with a scaly surface
> lumps.
> Lymphoma in the skin can look a lot like other skin conditions, such as eczema or psoriasis. Skin lymphomas are usually low-grade lymphomas. Sometimes other parts of the body are also affected but for most people with skin lymphoma, it stays in the skin.
> If you have a diagnosis of skin lymphoma and you are finding it hard to cope with your symptoms, there are some things you could try that might help. Also speak to your medical team for advice.
> **Contact your doctor urgently if you have a rash that starts suddenly and spreads quickly, a rash that is all over your body, or a rash with other symptoms such as pain, fever or breathlessness.**

➢ **Visit your GP if you have a rash that doesn't go away within a few days or that is interfering with your normal life.**

Brain and nerve symptoms

➢ Lymphoma that starts in or spreads to the brain or nervous system is very uncommon but can cause symptoms such as headaches, fits (seizures), memory problems, dizziness, sight problems, numbness, tingling or weakness in a limb. Many other conditions can also cause these symptoms, such as epilepsy, migraine or stroke.

Contact doctor if you have any of these symptoms.

➢ Swelling in the arms or legs
➢ Swollen lymph nodes can sometimes block the lymphatic vessels that run through the body. This stops fluid called lymph draining properly from the body's tissues. This fluid can build up, causing swelling and feelings of tightness, heaviness or soreness. This is called 'lymphoedema'. It usually affects an arm or a leg, although other areas of the body can be affected depending on where your lymphoma is. Other conditions, such as infection, injury, or some types of surgery, can also cause lymphoedema.
➢ It is important to know that lymphoedema is very uncommon and usually gets better once treatment

is started. If you are finding it hard to cope with, there are some things you can do that might help.

> **See a doctor for any symptoms of lymphoedema.**

Anaemia
> Around 1 in 3 people with lymphoma have anaemia (low number of red blood cells). This can make you feel tired and breathless because your body has to work harder than usual to get enough oxygen. You might look pale and you may have heart palpitations.
> Anaemia may be caused by lymphoma in the bone marrow or by bleeding due to lymphoma in the gut. If you have a swollen spleen, anaemia can also be caused by red blood cells collecting in the spleen or being destroyed in the spleen. Lots of other, less serious, conditions can also cause anaemia, such as heavy periods, pregnancy or stomach ulcers.

5 Coping with symptoms of lymphoma

This page has general advice and practical tips for coping with some of the common symptoms of lymphoma. We have a separate section on side effects of lymphoma treatment, which you might also find helpful.

Strong recommendations on managing symptoms.
> Coping with symptoms of lymphoma

- Coping with swollen lymph nodes
- Coping with fatigue
- Coping with weight loss
- Coping with night sweats
- Coping with itching
- Coping with pain
- Coping with skin symptoms
- Coping with swollen arms or legs
- Coping with your emotions

5.1 Coping with common symptoms of lymphoma

Coping with symptoms of lymphoma can be emotionally and physically challenging.

Suggestions to manage some of the more common symptoms.

5.2 Coping with swollen lymph nodes

I was very aware of a big node in my neck so I'd often wear a little scarf. I had another one under my arm and I would always wear something with sleeves because I was so aware of these big lumps and bumps.

Y, was diagnosed with small lymphocytic lymphoma in 2015

Swollen lymph nodes usually get better after treatment for lymphoma.

If you are on active monitoring (watch and wait), you are self-conscious about your lymph nodes, or you are finding it hard to cope with any change in your appearance, Macmillan has lots of resources that may help you.

It is natural to worry if you notice a new, or bigger, lymph node. Remember that it is normal for lymph nodes to go up and down over time. Lots of things – infections, skin conditions and immune diseases, for example – can cause lymph nodes to swell.

Checking your lymph nodes too frequently can cause unnecessary worry and also makes it more difficult to notice any changes in size of lymph nodes. Try not to check your nodes more than once a month.

You know your body and how you normally feel. If you notice any new, or bigger, lumps that last more than a week, contact your medical team.

5.3 Coping with fatigue

Fatigue is a common symptom of lymphoma and many people find it one of the hardest to live with. If you are struggling to cope with fatigue, speak to your medical team. They can check for any underlying conditions that might be making your fatigue worse (such as anaemia, depression or anxiety).

5.4 Coping with weight loss

If you have lost weight due to lymphoma and are now underweight, you can boost your energy (calorie) intake in the following ways:

- Choose full-fat options (for example, whole milk) over low-fat alternatives.
- Add cheese or sauces to pasta or vegetables.
- Add sugar, honey or syrup to drinks and puddings.
- Add butter or oil to bread, pasta, potatoes and vegetables.

Contact doctor if you lose more than 5% of your body weight over 6 to 12 months without trying to.

For example, if you normally weigh 10 stone, contact your doctor if you lose more than 7lbs.

5.5 Coping with night sweats

Night sweats can be caused by the lymphoma itself or by some treatments for lymphoma (for example, rituximab, and some chemotherapy drugs). For some women, certain types of chemotherapy may lead to menopause, which can also cause sweating. Some antidepressants can also cause night sweats.

If you are having treatment for your lymphoma, your night sweats often stop once you finish. However, they can sometimes carry on for a while. Here are a few suggestions that might help you cope with night sweats:

- **Keep your bedroom cool** – using a fan or keeping your window open might help. If you have a bedroom thermostat, try turning it down lower than usual.
- **Choose natural fabrics** such as cotton rather than man-made fabrics for bed sheets and your night clothes.
- **Use light layers** of nightclothes. This way you can take them off and put them back on easily.

- **Put a soft towel underneath you in bed** (some people put one on top too) to save your bed sheets from getting too wet.
- **Consider a mattress protector** or waterproof sheet. There are lots of options available in a variety of soft fabrics.
- **Make your bed in layers** if you often have to change your bedding in the night. Some people use a waterproof sheet and a normal sheet with another waterproof sheet and normal sheet on top. If the top layers get soaked through, it is easy to take them off in the middle of the night, leaving clean, dry bedding underneath.
- **Avoid spicy foods and sugary drinks**, especially in the evening.
- **Avoid alcohol and caffeinated drinks**.
- **Drink plenty of fluids** (2 to 3 litres a day, preferably cold drinks) to replace the fluids you lose through sweating.
- Exercise can help – earlier rather than later in the day.
- **Complementary therapy** and relaxation techniques, such as hypnosis or acupuncture, are helpful for some people.

5.6 Coping with itching

Itching due to lymphoma usually settles very quickly if you start treatment. However, it can be very troublesome, disrupting sleep and making it difficult to cope in the daytime. If it goes on for a long time, itching can lead to anxiety and depression and significantly reduce your quality of life.

If you are finding it hard to cope with itching, you might find the tips below helpful. If your itching is very intense or is interfering with your sleep or your day-to-day life, talk to your medical team. They may be able to prescribe medicine to help, such as:

- anti-histamines (for example, cetirizine or loratadine)
- antidepressants (for example, mirtazapine)
- medicines used to treat nerve pain (for example, carbamazepine or gabapentin)
- steroids (for example, prednisolone).

They might refer you for light therapy.

5.6.1 General tips

- **Try not to scratch** as you could be left with lasting scars. Instead, try rubbing in some cream, applying cool packs or pressing or tapping your fingers on your skin.
- **Cut your nails very short** to help prevent scratching.
- **Moisturise frequently throughout the day** with unscented moisturising creams or lotions or an anti-itch moisturiser, which your doctor or nurse can prescribe. Aim to moisturise two to three times a day and after bathing or showering. Try keeping your moisturiser in the fridge; the cooling effect can be soothing.
- **Make** time to relax – stress and anxiety can make itching worse and make it harder to cope. You may find relaxation and meditation techniques helpful.
- **Eat a** healthy diet **and drink plenty of water** – this can help to keep your skin hydrated and healthy.
- **Consider using a humidifier** to prevent your skin drying out.

5.6.2 Bathing and showering

- **Try not to bathe or shower too often** – the water can dry your skin and cause itching, so having short baths or showers may be better.
- **Use lukewarm water** – hot water can trigger itching.
- **Avoid bubble baths, perfumed soaps and perfumed shower gels**. If your skin isn't dirty, wash using plain water. If you need something more, try using a moisturising soap substitute (sometimes called an 'emollient wash product') or a skin cleanser designed for sensitive skin instead of soap. Your doctor might prescribe a product for you to use. Rinse your skin thoroughly to remove any residue.
- **Try taking an oatmeal bath**. This can be very soothing. You can buy oatmeal bath products or make your own by grinding uncooked, unflavoured oats to a very fine powder in a food processor or coffee grinder. Add about a cupful of the oatmeal powder to a lukewarm bath. The water should turn milky with a silky feel. Take care getting in and out of the bath as oatmeal will make it slippy.
- **Avoid scrubbing your skin** with a loofah, body puff or any type of body scrub. Try a soft, cotton washcloth instead.
- **Pat your skin dry** instead of rubbing it with a towel.
- **Avoid perfume or lanolin-based products** including perfumed deodorants and antiperspirants.
- **Avoid using alcohol-based products** such as wet wipes and antibacterial hand gel as these products can dry and irritate the skin.

5.6.3 Clothes

- **Wear loose-fitting clothing made of cotton** or other soft fabric, which is less itchy than wool or man-made fabrics.
- **Keep your night clothes and bed sheets light and loose** (again, cotton is better).
- **Wear cotton gloves at night** to stop you scratching during your sleep.
- **Avoid laundry detergent residue on clothing and bed sheets** – small traces of detergent can be left on clothes and make your skin itch. Try using a detergent that is made for washing babies' clothes as this will be softer on your skin. Give your washing an extra rinse at the end of the wash cycle.

5.7 Coping with pain

Lymphoma isn't usually painful but sometimes, swollen nodes press on other tissues and cause pain. This should improve if you have treatment.

Pain due to cancer can be managed. If you have pain due to lymphoma, tell your medical team. They can prescribe medicine to help.

Lots of different treatments are available. Your medical team will recommend the best option for you.

There are also things you can do yourself that might help you cope with your pain.

- **Take any pain medicine you have been prescribed** according to your doctor's instructions. It's important to realise that your body does not become immune to pain medicine. Don't wait until the pain gets unbearable before taking your medicine. This could make it harder to manage.

- **Try using heat to ease the pain**. You could use a hot water bottle, a microwaveable heat pack or a gel pad. Don't use them for longer than 10 minutes at a time and take care not to burn your skin. Hot baths and showers might also be soothing.
- **Try using an ice pack to numb the pain**. You can buy gel packs that go in the freezer or you can make your own from ice cubes or frozen peas. Make sure you wrap them in a towel to protect your skin. Again, limit their use to 10 minutes at a time and be careful not to damage your skin.
- **Relaxation techniques** such as meditation, imagery or mindfulness can be very helpful for some people. Consider complementary therapies such as acupuncture, massage, tai chi or yoga.

Do not use heat or ice packs over any area where circulation is poor.

5.8 Coping with skin symptoms

Skin (cutaneous) lymphoma is a rare condition with a variety of symptoms that can be distressing. Coping with swelling in the arms or legs

Lymphoedema (swelling in an arm or leg due to blocked lymphatic vessels) is uncommon in people with lymphoma and usually gets better after treatment. However, it can be very uncomfortable. It can also increase your risk of infection and blood clots.

If you have lymphoedema, your medical team might prescribe a 'gradient pressure garment' or 'lymphoedema stocking or sleeve'. This is a special type of elastic bandage that applies controlled pressure to the affected limb. It is tighter over your feet and hands than it is closer to your body to encourage the flow of lymphatic fluid.

There are also things you can do to help.

5.8.1 Skin care

- Keep your skin and nails clean and dry to help prevent infection.
- Moisturise your skin regularly.
- Use sunscreen to avoid getting sunburn.
- Cut your toenails straight across rather than in a curved shape to prevent ingrowing toenails and infections.
- If you need to check the temperature of the bath, use the unaffected arm or leg.
- Use a thimble if you do any needlework.

5.8.2 Healthcare

- Make sure any blood tests, blood pressure measurements or injections you need are in the unaffected arm.
- Be aware of the signs of infection.

5.8.3 Clothing

- Wear loose-fitting clothes and jewellery and cotton socks.
- Avoid going outside in bare feet.
- Wear gloves for gardening and cooking.

5.8.4 Lifestyle

- Keep the affected arm or leg elevated whenever possible.

- Try to avoid putting pressure on the affected arm or leg.
- If your legs are affected, do not sit with your legs crossed.
- Don't sit in the same position for more than 30 minutes at a time.
- Don't use heat packs on the affected arm or leg. This could increase blood flow and make the swelling worse.
- Exercise can improve the lymphatic drainage from the affected limb.

5.9 Coping with your emotions

If you are struggling with your feelings, you might find it helpful to visit our page on the emotional impact of lymphoma. We have some suggestions on how to cope with difficult feelings.

6 Tests, diagnosis and staging

Doctors use tests and scans to diagnose lymphoma and to find out more about it after a diagnosis is confirmed. This helps them plan the best treatment for you.

You continue to have tests and scans during treatment, follow-up and any periods of 'watch and wait'.

This section outlines the referral process and the tests and scans you might have at hospital.

6.1 Getting a referral for tests

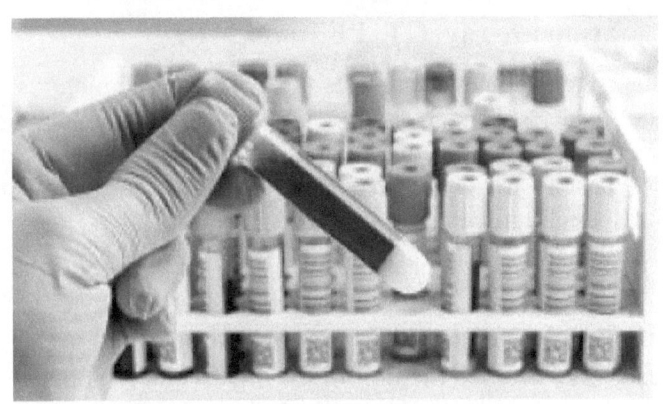

6.2 Blood tests

Blood tests show how your body is affected by lymphoma and tell doctors about your general health.

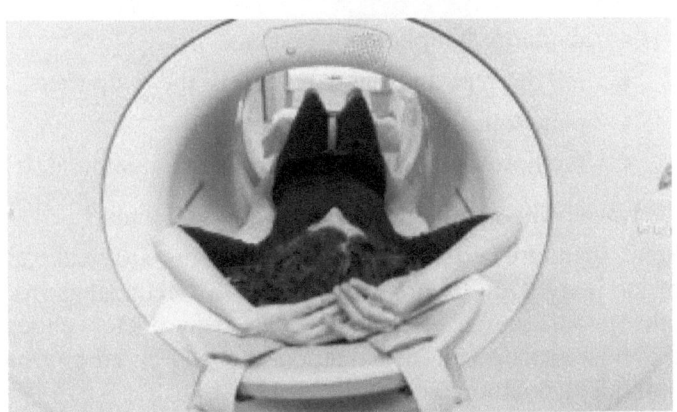

6.3 X-ray, CT, MRI, and PET scans

7 Scans: X-ray, CT, PET and MRI

This page is about scans, tests that take detailed pictures of the inside of your body. The results give doctors information about your lymphoma and help them decide how best to treat you. We have separate information on ultrasound scans.

7.1 Overview of scans

7.1.1 What is a scan?

Scans give detailed pictures of the organs and lymph nodes (glands) in your body. There are different types of scan that work in different ways.

7.1.2 What are scans used for?

Depending on the type of scan, the results may help your doctors to:

- diagnose lymphoma
- tell the type and stage (extent) of the lymphoma
- plan your treatment
- see how well you have responded to treatment.

7.1.3 Why are there different types of scans?

Some scans are better than others at checking different parts of the body. Don't worry if you have different scans from other people you meet at the hospital – your doctors choose the most appropriate investigations for you based on your individual situation?

7.1.4 What is a contrast agent?

You might be given a contrast agent before your scan. This is a type of dye. It helps to show internal structures (blood vessels, organs and tissues) clearly.

Depending on the part of your body being scanned, you have a contrast agent either as:

- a drink
- an injection into a vein in your arm.

If you have a contrast agent, there is a small risk that you could have an allergic reaction. Hospital staff are well-trained in dealing with this.

7.1.5 Are scans safe?

Scans are generally considered to be safe, although some scans do use radiation. Doctors weigh the risks of any scan against the benefits.

Ionising radiation can be harmful to DNA (genetic material in our cells). It is thought that it could very slightly increase your risk of developing cancer in the future. However, the amount of radiation you are exposed to during a scan is carefully controlled to keep it as low as possible. This minimises any risks. Who carries out scans?

The scans on this page will be carried out by a radiographer, a specialist in using equipment to diagnose and treat people who are unwell.

7.2 What is an X-ray scan?

An X-ray scan, usually just referred to as an X-ray, takes pictures of the inside of your body. X-ray scans use ionising (high-energy) radiation to make pictures from the front to the back of your body.

On the scan image:

- bone and contrast agent appears as white
- air (for example in the chest) appears as black
- muscle, fat and fluid appear in shades of grey.

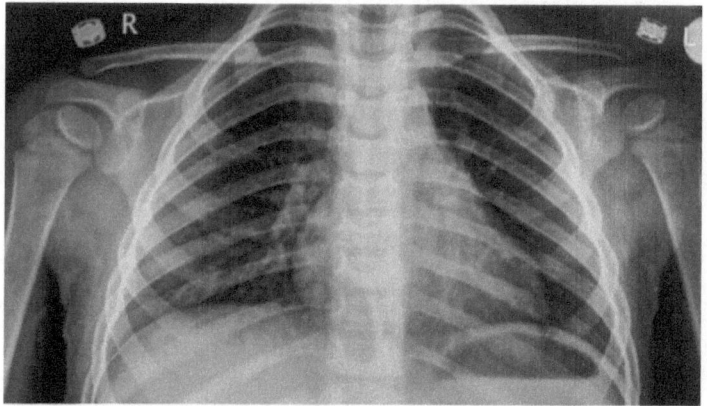

Figure: A chest X-Ray

Lymphoma is sometimes first picked up on an X-ray, for example on:

- a chest X-ray done to find out why you are short of breath or have a cough
- an abdominal X-ray if you have pain in your tummy or a change of bowel habit such as diarrhoea.

If you have a central line to give you chemotherapy, you might have an X-ray to check the position of it.

You may have an X-ray later on, too, for example, to find out if any new symptoms are due to infection or treatment side effects.

7.3 What is the process for having an X-ray scan?

X-ray scans are usually done as an outpatient procedure, which means that you don't have to stay in hospital overnight. You should be able to have your X-ray at your local hospital.

X-ray scans take around 15 minutes for a simple ('plain') X-ray. The scan is not painful.

7.3.1 How should I prepare?

You should be given information about how to prepare for the scan.

You can eat and drink as normal on the day of your scan. It is safe to continue taking any prescription medication on the day of your appointment.

You are then asked to take off any metal you are wearing (for example, jewellery, a belt, your watch, an underwired bra). If you wear glasses, you might be asked to remove them.

When you attend your appointment, staff in the scanning department ask if you are pregnant or could be pregnant.

7.3.2 What happens during the procedure?

An X-ray machine looks like a tube and has a light bulb at one end. You may have the X-rays taken while you are standing, or while you are sitting or lying down on a couch. You are not closed in during the scan.

The radiographer checks that that you are in the right position. To do this, they might gently press on some parts of your body.

During the scan, the radiographer stands behind a screen.

You need to be very still while the pictures are taken. You might be asked to hold your breath for a few seconds during the scan to reduce movement and blurring of the images.

7.3.3 What happens after the procedure?

You can go straight home after having an X-ray scan. There are no precautions you need to take afterwards.

7.4 What is a computed tomography (CT) scan?

A computed tomography (CT) scan uses a type of X-ray. The scan shows detailed cross-sectional images of the inside of your body. It also shows up areas of disease (such as swollen lymph nodes) more clearly than plain X-rays do.

A CT scan takes a number of narrow X-rays, like 'slices' through the body. The images are analysed by a computer and put back together to form a very detailed 3D (three-dimensional) picture of your organs.

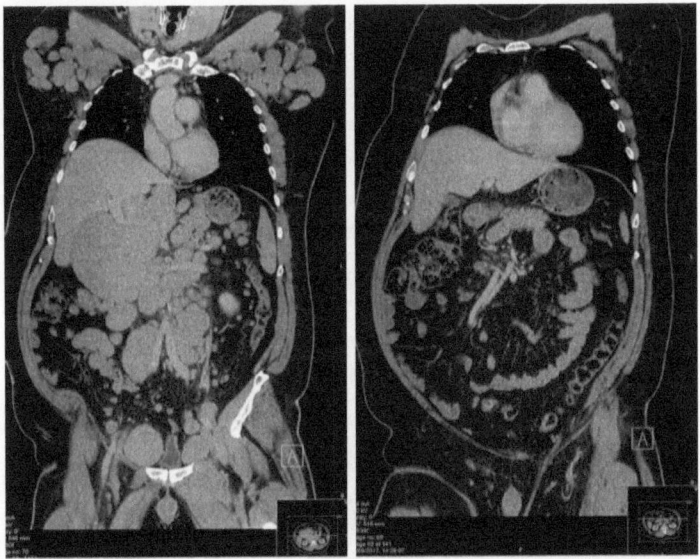

Figure Left: Enlarged lymph nodes (swollen glands) in armpits and abdomen (tummy) on a CT scan at diagnosis

Figure Right: Subsequent good quality response to treatment

CT scans are used to look at the head and neck, spine, chest, abdomen (stomach) and pelvis. They are used:

- to diagnose and stage lymphoma
- to perform CT guided biopsy – for example in the abdomen or chest, if needed
- as part of radiotherapy planning

- to check your response to treatment by comparing scans taken before, during and at the end of a course of treatment.

7.5 What is the process for having a CT scan?

CT scans are usually done as an outpatient procedure, which means that you don't have to stay in hospital overnight. You should be able to have your CT scan at your local hospital.

CT scans take around 45 minutes and are not painful. Due to this length of time, you may be asked to empty your bladder beforehand.

If you feel anxious about any aspect of having a scan, speak to your medical team.

7.5.1 How should I prepare?

You should be given information about how to prepare for the scan.

You might be told not to eat for a couple of hours before your scan.

It is generally safe to continue taking any prescription medication on the day of your appointment. However, you may not be able to take certain types of medication for diabetes on the day. You will be given advice by the CT scanning department about when to take your tablets or insulin.

When you attend your appointment, staff in the scanning department ask if you are pregnant or could be pregnant.

You will also be asked if have asthma or diabetes. If you do, the hospital will carry out a thorough assessment. They will then decide on a course of action that is appropriate to your situation.

Before your scan, you may also be given a contrast agent (dye). However, you will first be asked if you have ever had an allergic reaction to a contrast agent.

You are then asked to take off any metal you are wearing (for example, jewellery, a belt, your watch, an underwired bra). If you wear glasses, you might be asked to remove them.

7.5.2 What happens during the procedure?

The CT scanner is a large cylinder with a couch in the middle of it – it looks a bit like a doughnut. Usually, you lie on your back on the couch, which moves you slowly into the scanner.

You need to lie very still while the scan pictures are taken. You might be asked to hold your breath for approximately 6 seconds during the scan. This reduces your movement and therefore blurring of the scan images.

You are alone in the scanning room during the scan itself. Staff can see you all the time through a glass window and a video camera, and they can talk to you. You can alert them if you feel unwell or distressed – you can ask for help or raise a hand.

Some people worry about feeling claustrophobic (closed in). However, the scanning machine does not surround your whole body at any one time and the scan is also quick (taking under than around 30 seconds), so most people find it okay

7.5.3 What happens after the procedure?

You can usually go straight home after your scan.

7.6 What is a positron-emission tomography (PET) scan?

PET scans, like CT scans, can help doctors work out which parts of your body are involved by lymphoma and which are not.

A positron-emission tomography (PET) scan uses a radiotracer or 'tracer' (radioactive form of sugar) to show up the most active cells in your body. In some types of lymphoma, the cells are very active so show up clearly on a PET scan.

The radiotracer that is usually used is fluoro-deoxy-glucose (FDG). You are given this by injection into a vein before you have the scan. The FDG travels to the cells in the body that use glucose (a sugar) for energy. Cancerous (including lymphoma) cells use up a lot of energy and so need a lot of glucose. The radiotracer is taken up into these cancerous cells and becomes trapped there. These cells then show up as 'hot spots' on the scan.

You may have a CT scan at the same appointment. This is known as a PET/CT scan.

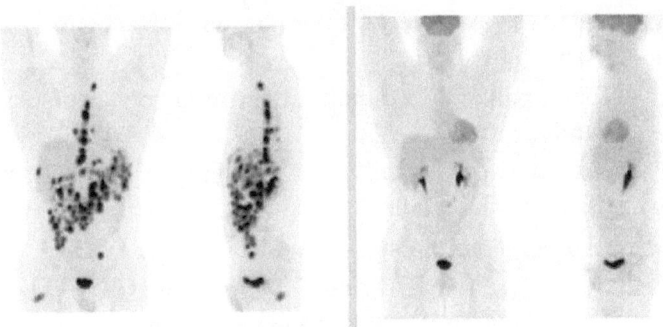

Figure Left: Non-Hodgkin lymphoma stage IV. Figure Right: Complete response to treatment

PET scans can be used:
- before treatment to stage the lymphoma
- after a few cycles of treatment, to help doctors plan further treatment
- after a course of treatment, to see how well you have responded to it
- to assess your lymphoma if your medical team are considering changing your treatment
- to find our if your lymphoma has relapsed (come back), if your symptoms have returned or new ones begun.

Note: if you need a PET scan after a course of treatment, you will usually not have one straightaway. There might still be some inflammation (swelling) where the lymphoma was, which could confuse the results. Radiologists usually recommend waiting:

- at least 3–4 weeks after the end of a course of chemotherapy.
- approximately 3 months after the end of a course of radiotherapy.

PET scans are most useful when the lymphoma cells are very active, which includes:

- Hodgkin lymphoma
- high-grade non-Hodgkin lymphomas such as diffuse large B-cell lymphoma, Burkitt lymphoma, lymphoblastic lymphoma.

7.7 What is the process for having a PET scan?

Most of the time, a PET scan is done together with a CT scan. This is known as a PET/CT scan. Combining the images from both scans gives a much clearer picture of exactly which areas of your body are affected by the lymphoma.

PET scans are usually done as an outpatient procedure, which means that you don't have to stay in hospital overnight. Not all hospitals have a PET scanning machine so you might have to travel to a larger centre to have your scan. Otherwise, you may be able to have one at a mobile unit.

PET scans often take around 30–60 minutes. Due to this length of time, you may be asked to empty your bladder beforehand.

The scan is not painful, but you might find it uncomfortable to lie still for a long time. If you think you are likely to find this difficult, ask your doctor for advice about how to cope with the discomfort. You might need to take relief medication beforehand.

The PET scan itself takes less than an hour, but you are usually in the scanning department for around 2–3 hours in total.

7.7.1 How should I prepare?

You will be given information about how to prepare for the scan.

It is advisable to wear something that will keep you warm during the scan.

For around 4–6 hours before your scan, you can only drink plain water (although sometimes black coffee or tea is allowed – check with the hospital staff).

It is generally safe to continue taking any prescription medication on the day of your appointment. However, if you are on medication for diabetes, you cannot take medication for diabetes on the day. You will be given advice about when to take your tablets or insulin.

Do not take strenuous exercise in the 6 hours before the scan; this can cause your muscles to take up the glucose radiotracer and could confuse the results.

Before your appointment, let the hospital staff know if you are:

- pregnant, or could be pregnant
- breastfeeding
- diabetic and how your diabetes is being treated – you should be given advice about eating and about when to take your tablets or insulin before the scan.

Before your scan, you may be given a contrast agent (dye).

You are then asked to take off any metal you are wearing (for example jewellery, a belt, your watch, an underwired bra). If you wear glasses, you might be asked to remove them.

You then have your blood sugar levels checked, usually through a finger prick test. A cannula (small tube) is then put into a vein, typically in your arm. The cannula is used to give you the radiotracer injection.

You might be given a contrast agent as a drink.

After you have been given the radiotracer, you have to sit or lie down to relax in a quiet, dimly lit place for at least an hour before you have the scan. This gives enough time for the radiotracer to travel through your body. Due to the length of time you may have to lie still for, you will usually be asked to empty your bladder before the scan.

7.7.2 What happens during the procedure?

The PET scanner is a large cylinder with a couch in the middle of it – it looks a bit like a doughnut.

You are asked to keep as still as possible during the scan. Although the scan itself is not painful, you might be uncomfortable, especially if you have to keep your arms above your head.

You are alone in the scanning room during the scan. The hospital staff will be behind a glass screen and can also see you via video camera. You are able to speak to them and they can speak to you via a two-way speaker.

Some people worry about feeling claustrophobic (closed in). However, the scanning machine does not surround your whole body at any one time so most people find it okay.

What happens after the procedure?

You can usually go straight home after your scan.

Note: you should avoid close contact with pregnant women, babies and young children for 6 hours after your PET scan. This is because you still have some radioactivity in your body from the radiotracer. It should mostly leave your body after about 6 hours.

Airports often have radiation alarms that you could set off. If you travel by plane within a few days, you could take your scan appointment letter to show that you have recently had a scan.

7.8 What is a magnetic resonance imaging (MRI) scan?

A magnetic resonance imaging (MRI) scan uses magnets and radio waves to make detailed cross-sectional images of the inside of your body.

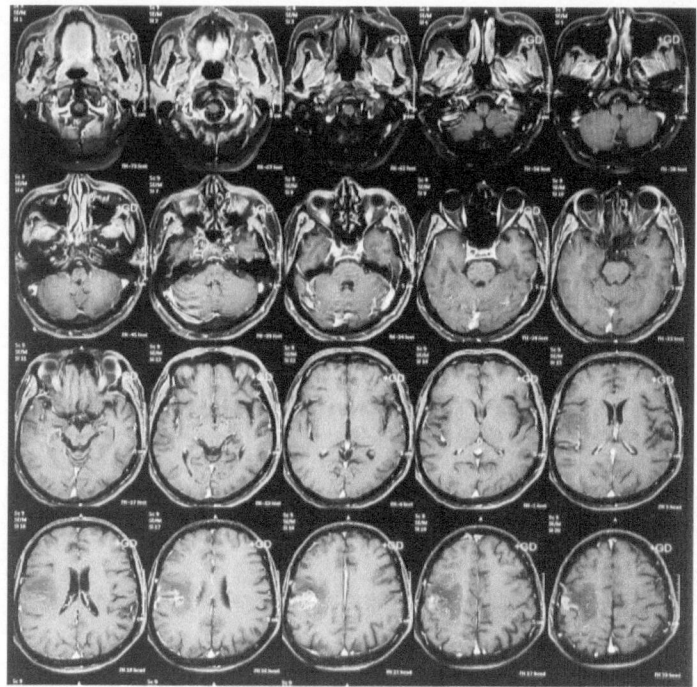

Figure: An MRI scan showing images of the brain

You might have an MRI scan to:
- diagnose and assess lymphomas of the central nervous system (brain and spinal cord) or the head and neck.

You might have an MRI instead of a CT or PET/CT scan if:
- you are allergic to contrast agents, which are often used in CT and PET/CT scans
- you are pregnant.

7.9 What is the process for having an MRI scan?

MRI scans are usually done as an outpatient procedure, which means that you don't have to stay in hospital overnight. Not all hospitals have an MRI scanning machine. You might have to travel to a larger hospital to have your scan.

MRI scans can take anywhere from 30 minutes to over an hour. Due to this length of time, you may be asked to empty your bladder beforehand.

The scan is not painful, but you might find it uncomfortable to lie still for a long time.

7.9.1 How should I prepare?

You should be given information about how to prepare for the scan.

You can usually eat and drink as normal on the day of your scan. Depending on which part of your body is being scanned, though, you may be advised not to eat or drink for up to 4 hours before your scan. Or you might be told to drink a large amount of water beforehand.

It is generally safe to continue taking any prescription medication on the day of your appointment. If you are on medication for diabetes, you will be given advice about when to take your tablets or insulin.

You must:

- tell the staff if you have any metal in your body, such as staples from previous surgery, metal plates put in after an injury, a hip replacement or a pacemaker

- take off metal (for example, jewellery, a belt, your watch, an underwired bra, glasses).

You may be given a contrast agent (dye).

If you have an MRI scan of your brain, you might be given a contrast agent. You should be asked if you have any allergies, kidney problems or problems with blood clotting before you have this contrast agent. This is so that hospital staff can take any necessary precautions.

When you attend your appointment, staff in the scanning department ask if you:

- are pregnant, or could be pregnant
- have any implants in your body, especially those containing iron (for example a hip replacement or pacemaker). You will not have an MRI scan if the metal is not compliant with the MRI scanner.
- have ever had an allergic reaction to a contrast agent.

7.9.2 What happens during the procedure?

The MRI scanner is a large cylinder with a couch in the middle of it – it looks a bit like a doughnut. The cylinder measures radio waves as they pass through your body.

The couch moves you into the scanner. You are asked to keep as still as possible during the scan. You might find it uncomfortable to lie still for as long as is needed – if you think you are likely to find this difficult, ask your doctor for advice about how to cope with the discomfort. You might need to take pain relief medication beforehand.

Being in an MRI scanner can feel hot and can be very noisy. You might also feel vibrations and slight movement of the couch during the scan. You should be offered earplugs or you may be able to listen to music during the scan.

You might feel enclosed inside an MRI scanner. Some people feel claustrophobic (closed in). There will be a two-way speaker in the machine so that you can hear and speak to the radiographers. You will also have a buzzer to use if you want to let the staff know you feel distressed. If you feel anxious about having your scan, speak to a member of hospital staff.

7.9.3 What happens after the procedure?

You can usually go straight home after your scan, though you shouldn't drive if you have had a sedative or a contrast agent.

7.10 Frequently asked questions about scans

7.10.1 Can I have a scan if I am pregnant or breastfeeding?

The advice on scans during pregnancy and while breastfeeding depends on the type of scan you have.

X-ray scans

There is a small risk of an unborn baby being exposed to radiation during an X-ray scan. This could increase their risk of developing cancer in childhood. However, most X-ray scans use a low dosage of radiation, so the risks are very small.

Doctors carefully assess the risks and benefits of giving people who are pregnant an X-ray scan. If an X-ray scan is considered to be necessary, they will protect your baby using lead shielding during the scan.

Breastfeeding is generally considered to be safe after an X-ray scan.

CT scans

There is a small risk to an unborn baby from a CT scan, especially during the first trimester of pregnancy. If you are pregnant, you may have a different type of scan to assess the lymphoma, for example an ultrasound scan or a magnetic resonance imaging (MRI) scan.

Breastfeeding is generally considered to be safe after a CT scan (including if you have had a contrast agent). However, you may be advised not to breastfeed for a day or two afterwards. Follow the advice of your doctors.

PET scans

PET scans cause a risk to an unborn baby. If you are pregnant, your doctor might advise that you have a different type of scan to assess the lymphoma, for example a magnetic resonance imaging (MRI) scan.

If you are breastfeeding, you might be advised to stop for a while after having the radiotracer injection. Follow the advice of your doctors.

MRI scans

There is no evidence that MRI scans are unsafe during pregnancy. However, doctors often avoid giving this type of scan during the first trimester when the baby's organs are developing.

The contrast agent used in MRI scans enters the breast milk only in extremely small amounts. Breastfeeding therefore does not put your baby at risk.

7.10.2 Are scans painful?

Scans are not painful but you may find it uncomfortable if you need to still for a long time. Hospitals often have a range of supports to help keep you comfortable.

If you think you are likely to find it difficult to lie still for the time, ask your doctor for advice about how to cope with the discomfort. You might need to take pain relief medication beforehand.

7.10.3 Do scans use radiation?

Some scans use radiation. This includes X-ray scans, CT scans, PET scans and PET/CT scans. MRI scans do not use radiation.

Radiation is a type of energy. We are exposed to low levels of radiation every day. There are two types of radiation:

- non-ionising (low energy), which comes from natural sources such as soil and water
- ionising (high energy), which is man-made. This is the type of radiation used in some cancer treatments. It works by making breaks in the DNA (genetic material) in cells.

Ionising radiation can cause cancer. However, the levels you are exposed to during medical tests and scans are carefully controlled and kept as low as possible. This means that the risk it poses is very low.

7.10.4 Will I be radioactive after a scan?

Being radioactive means giving off radiation. Whether you are radioactive for a short while after your scan depends on the type of scan you have.

You will not be radioactive after:

- an X-ray scan
- a CT scan
- an MRI scan

After a PET or a PET/CT scan, you will be radioactive for around 6 hours. You should avoid being around women who are pregnant during this time.

7.10.5 Are there any side effects of having a contrast agent?

The contrast agent during a CT scan might make you feel hot all over, but this usually only lasts for a few minutes. Sometimes people feel sick after the contrast agent.

If you have a contrast agent by injection, it can sometimes sting and may make you feel warm or cold where the contrast is injected. With an iodine contrast agent injected into your arm, you may feel a warm sensation travelling down your arms. This tends to pass very quickly.

Other common and short-lasting sensations with an iodine contrast agent injection include:

- a strange taste in your mouth
- feeling as though you are passing urine.

A small number of people have an allergic reaction to the contrast agent. This can cause itchy skin, swollen lumps in the skin. Very rarely, contrast agents cause a more serious allergic reaction, leading to breathing problems and swelling of the throat. Hospital staff are trained to treat any allergic reactions that develop.

You might be asked to arrive at your appointment an hour early. You will be asked if you have ever had an allergic reaction to a contrast agent before. You'll also be asked other questions about your general health to check that it is safe for you to have the contrast agent. In some departments, you may be asked to stay in the hospital for a short time after a CT scan if you have had intravenous contrast. This allows time for hospital staff to check for any signs of an allergic reaction.

7.10.6 When will I get the results?

Your doctor usually gets the results from the hospital within a few days and will discuss them with you. Staff in the scanning department won't be able to give you your scan results while you are at the hospital.

7.10.7 I feel anxious about having the scan – what can I do?

Talk to the staff in scanning department at your hospital if you are worried about any part of having your scan. They can answer any questions you have and may be able to suggest ways of coping with your anxiety.

If you feel very anxious, you may be able to have an anti-anxiety drug before your scan. This is more common with MRI than with other types of scan. If you feel an anti-anxiety drug could help you, talk to the staff in the scanning department about this possibility in advance of your appointment.

Some people find that listening to a CD during the scan helps to take their mind off of the procedure. You could ask your hospital if you are able to take someone with you to your appointment.

For some people, waiting for test results can be a particularly anxious time. Although the wait might feel long, it is important that doctors collect all of the information they need in order to plan the best treatment for you.

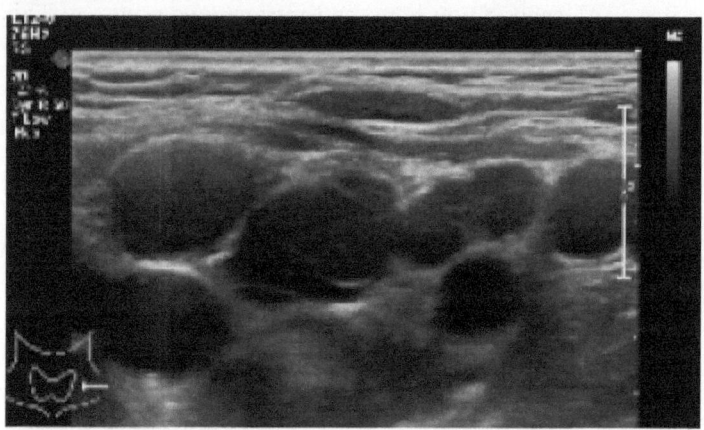

7.11 Ultrasound scan

These scans use sound waves to take pictures of the inside of your body.

8 Ultrasound scan

An ultrasound scan uses sound waves to make pictures of the inside of your body. It can help doctors diagnose and find out information about some types of lymphoma.

8.1 What is an ultrasound scan?

An ultrasound scan makes pictures of the inside of your body. Ultrasound scans use sound waves. The sound waves come out of an instrument called a 'probe' and travel through your body. They are very high-frequency (fast-travelling) so you cannot hear them. The waves bounce off of your tissues and organs. The echoes create a picture of the inside of your body.

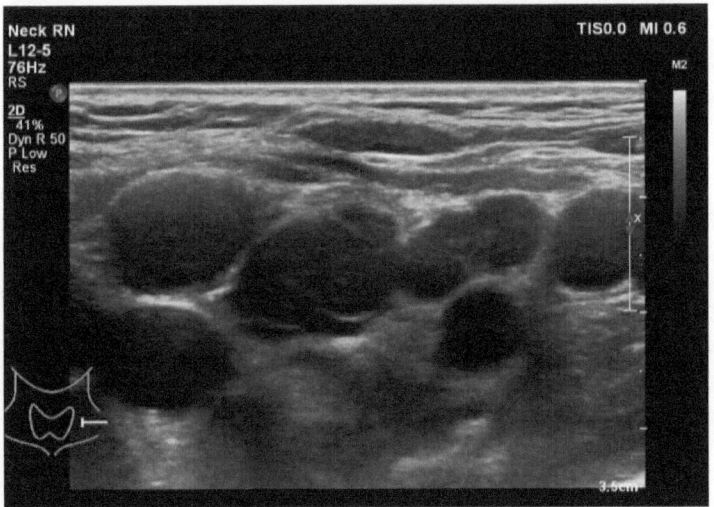

Figure: Ultrasound image showing lymph nodes (glands) in the neck.

Ultrasound is used in people with lymphoma to:

- examine the neck, the organs in the abdomen (stomach) or the pelvis. It might also be used to examine other sites (areas) of swelling such as under the armpits or in the groin area.
- help find the best place to biopsy a lymph node (gland) or other swelling (ultrasound-guided biopsy).

- help find the best position for putting in a central line (thin tube put into a vein to give you drugs and to take blood samples).

In a small number of people affected by lymphoma who require drainage of fluid, ultrasound may be used to guide this process.

8.2 What is the process for having an ultrasound scan?

Ultrasound scans are usually done as an outpatient procedure, which means that you don't have to stay in hospital overnight.

Ultrasound scans take around 15 minutes and are not painful.

8.2.1 How do I prepare for an ultrasound scan?

You should be given information about how to prepare for the scan.

You should be told in advance if you need to have a full or an empty bladder for the scan. You may also be advised not to eat anything for a few hours beforehand.

8.2.2 What happens during the procedure?

The procedure depends on which type of ultrasound scan you have:

- an external ultrasound scan uses a probe over your skin
- an internal ultrasound scan inserts a probe into your body.

External ultrasound scan
You might have an external ultrasound scan to examine lumps that are palpable (can be felt) in areas such as your:

- abdomen (if you have abdominal pain)
- arms
- armpit
- groin
- legs
- neck.

A radiographer or a sonographer (specialists in medical imagery and diagnostics) rubs gel onto the skin over the part of your body that they want to examine. They then gently press a hand-held probe (which looks a bit like a microphone) onto your skin. They move it around to make a picture on a computer screen. This type of ultrasound scan takes about 15 minutes.

Internal ultrasound scan
Internal ultrasound scans are not frequently used in lymphoma.

An internal ultrasound uses a tiny camera to look at your organs. The camera is attached either to a probe or to an endoscope (flexible tube). This is passed into an opening in your body (usually your mouth).

You might be given a sedative (relaxant) to make the procedure easier and more comfortable.

This type of ultrasound takes a bit longer.

8.2.3 What happens after the procedure?

You can go straight home after your scan, though you won't be able to drive if you have had a sedative.

Ultrasound scans do not use radiation. There are no precautions you need to take afterwards.

8.3 Frequently asked questions about ultrasound scans

8.3.1 Do I need to fast (not eat or drink) on the day of the scan?

You may be advised not to eat for a few hours before your scan.

8.3.2 Is it Okay to take prescription medication before the scan?

It is generally safe to continue taking any prescription medication on the day of your appointment. Check with hospital staff, though, and follow their advice.

8.3.3 Will I be closed in during the scan?

You will not be closed in during the scan – you will lie down on a couch.

If you feel anxious about having your scan, speak to your medical team.

8.3.4 When will I get the results?

Your doctor usually gets the results from the hospital within a few days and will discuss them with you. Staff in the scanning department won't be able to give you your scan results while you are at the hospital.

8.3.5 Are ultrasound scans safe?

Ultrasound scans are very safe. They do not use any radiation.

8.3.6 Can I have an ultrasound scan if I am pregnant or breastfeeding?

There are no known risks to an unborn baby from an ultrasound scan. Breastfeeding is also considered to be safe after an ultrasound scan.

8.4 What if I feel anxious about having the scan?

For some people, waiting for test results can be a particularly anxious time. Although the wait might feel long, it is important that doctors collect all of the information they need in order to plan the best treatment for you.

Talk to the staff in the scanning department at your hospital if you are worried about having your scan. They can answer any questions you have and may be able to suggest ways of coping with your anxiety.

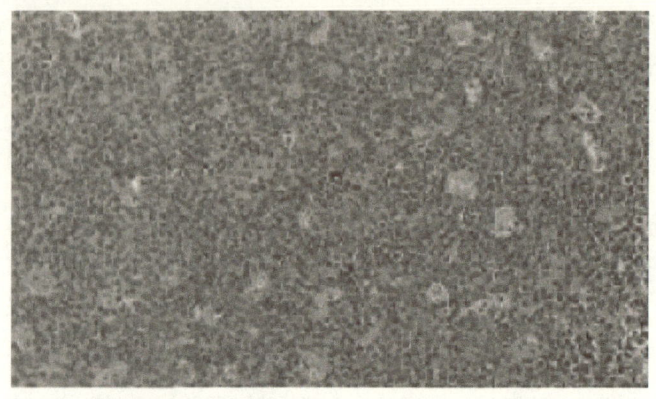

8.5 Biopsy

A biopsy (sample of tissue) is usually needed before a diagnosis of lymphoma can be confirmed.

9 Biopsy

A biopsy is a sample of tissue taken from your body that is then looked at under a microscope to check for abnormal cells. In most cases, a biopsy is the only way to confirm a diagnosis of lymphoma.

9.1 What is a biopsy?

A biopsy is a medical procedure that takes a sample of tissue from your body to be examined in a laboratory. The tissue sample itself may also be called a 'biopsy' or a 'biopsy sample'.

The laboratory may use special stains (dyes) or do tests on the tissue. A histopathologist looks at the slides to check for abnormal cells to see if lymphoma is present.

To diagnose lymphoma, a biopsy sample is often taken from a lymph node. Lymph nodes are part of the immune system. Lymph nodes are small, oval swellings arranged in groups at various points along the lymphatic drainage system, for example, in the neck, armpit, groin, chest and abdomen. They help fight infections and drain waste fluids from the body's tissues.

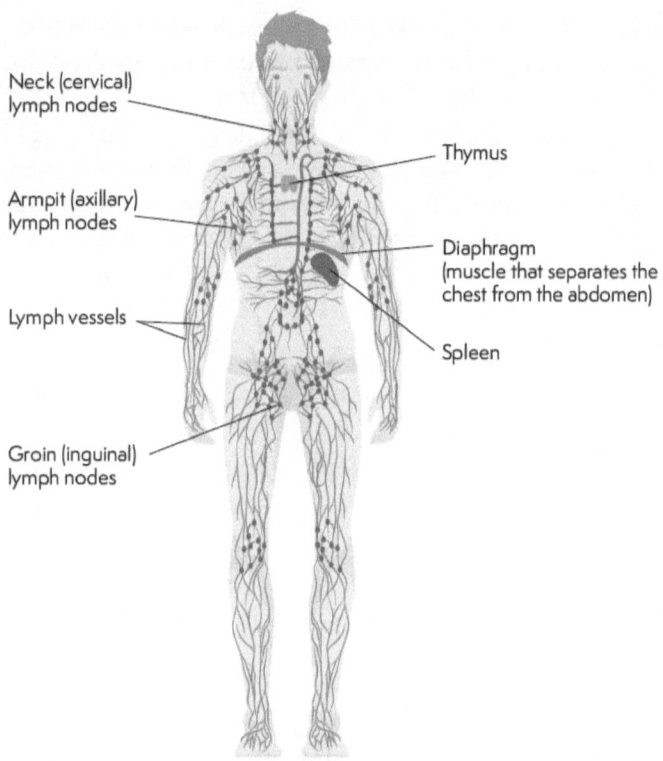

Figure: The lymphatic system

9.2 Why might I need a biopsy?

A biopsy is usually the only way to confirm lymphoma. Your doctor might also ask you to have a biopsy to:

- tell which type the lymphoma is
- monitor whether your lymphoma is growing and when to begin treatment

- check how well your lymphoma has responded to the treatment.

9.3 What are the different types of biopsy?

There are several types of biopsy, including:

- excision biopsy, where a lymph node (gland) is completely removed
- incisional biopsy, where part of a lymph node is removed
- core needle biopsy, where a small sample of the lymph node is taken (also known as a 'core biopsy' or a 'needle biopsy')
- laparoscopic (keyhole) biopsy, where all or part of a lymph node is removed.

All of these procedures are safe and well-established.

9.3.1 Excision biopsy

Excision biopsy is the most common type of biopsy used to diagnose lymphoma. This procedure removes a whole lymph node, giving doctors a large enough sample to tell whether or not lymphoma is present. Additional tests can be done on the tissue sample, should they be needed.

Excision biopsy is a minor operation. You go to hospital as an outpatient and the visit takes a few hours.

The procedure is performed under local or general anaesthetic. If the lymph node is near the surface of your skin, you usually have a local anaesthetic. If it is deeper inside your body, you might have a general anaesthetic.

Imaging scans (such as a CT, ultrasound, X-ray or MRI) are sometimes done before an excision biopsy. These images help to guide your surgeon to the exact place to take the biopsy sample from. After the scan, the area is cleaned and numbed it. The surgeon removes the lymph node and sends the tissue to a laboratory where it is examined by a pathologist.

After an excision biopsy, your wound is stitched and dressed. You should be given information about how to care for the biopsied area. If you are not offered this advice, ask for it.

You are allowed to go home as soon as you can pass urine and walk. It is not safe for you to drive yourself home if you had a general anaesthetic. You may be able to drive if you had local anaesthetic but it is usually advised to have someone collect you from the hospital.

Stitches are normally removed a week later, either at your doctor or at the hospital.

9.3.2 Incisional biopsy

Incisional biopsy is commonly used in cases where lymph nodes are large. The procedure is similar to that of an excisional biopsy, but only part (as opposed to all) of a lymph node is removed.

9.3.3 Core needle biopsy

Core needle biopsy takes a small sample of the lymph node. Your doctor might do a core needle biopsy if there is a possibility that the node is swollen because of an infection or because of cancer that has spread from elsewhere in your body. Core needle biopsy might also be recommended when it is too difficult to remove the whole gland. Your doctor may still ask you to have an excision biopsy at a later date, particularly, if the core needle biopsy sample is not large enough to rule out lymphoma.

Core needle biopsy is a minor procedure. Usually, it takes around 15–30 minutes. It is usually performed under local anaesthetic. A surgeon or radiologist uses a hollow needle to remove some of the tissue from the lymph node before sending it to a laboratory for examination.

If the lymph node to be biopsied is near to the surface of your skin, the surgeon can feel for it. If it is deeper within your body, they might ask you to have an ultrasound or CT scan, performed by a radiologist. The scan images help guide the doctor to the exact place to take the biopsy sample from.

After a core biopsy, your wound is dressed. You should be given information about how to care for the biopsied area. If you are not offered this advice, ask for it. You can go home soon after your biopsy; occasionally, you may be asked to stay in the day ward for a few hours of observation afterwards. It is generally safe for you to drive yourself home.

9.3.4 Laparoscopic (keyhole) biopsy

Laparoscopic (keyhole) biopsy involves a surgeon making a small incision (cut) through your skin. A very narrow instrument is then passed through the incision and all or part of a lymph node is removed.

You might have a laparoscopic biopsy if the lymph nodes affected are deep within your body, for example, in your abdomen (tummy).

Laparoscopic biopsy is performed under general anaesthetic. You might need to stay in hospital overnight, but you should be allowed to go home the next day. It may be safe for you to drive but it is advisable to have someone collect you.

After a laparoscopic biopsy, your wound is dressed. You should be given information about how to care for the biopsied area. If you are not offered this advice, ask for it.

9.4 How should I care for the biopsied area?

After your biopsy, a medical professional checks that it is safe for you to go home. They put a protective dressing on the area where the biopsy was taken from. Most dressings are waterproof, though they may not withstand a power shower (which gives a high pressure water spray). Your medical team should give you clear guidance on how to care for the biopsied area.

Below is some general guidance about how to care for the biopsied area. Always follow the specific advice given to you by your doctor or nurse.

- Leave the dressing on for a few days.
- Avoid swimming pools, saunas, hot tubs and Jacuzzis until the wound is healed (which usually takes around 7–10 days).

Note: Seek medical advice straightaway if you notice signs of infection, including bleeding, swelling of or discharge from the biopsied area, fever (a temperature above 38°C), chills and sweating.

9.4.1 How long does it take to recover after a biopsy?

It can take up to a couple of weeks for any swelling, soreness and bruising to go down after a biopsy. During this time, follow the advice given to you by the hospital about how to care for the biopsied area. While the area is healing, you may need to avoid strenuous exercise and heavy lifting.

9.5 How long does it take for results to come back?

The length of time it takes for your results to come back depends on the practice at your hospital and on your circumstances. Ask your doctor what to expect. Sometimes results come through within a few days; other times they take around a week. Your biopsy sample may need to be sent away for further laboratory tests, in which case the result may take longer.

Lymphoma is a complex disease. Special stains are often needed to look at the biopsy slides. It is also not uncommon for pathologists to consult with a colleague. Your medical team will talk to you about specific treatment as soon as they are satisfied that they have a firm diagnosis. In the meantime, it is possible to get ahead with staging tests and other assessments. Your team can also talk to you in general terms about treatment types.

It is natural to feel anxious while you are waiting for your results. Contact your doctor if you are concerned about the length of time you have been waiting

9.6 Will I need further tests?

Further biopsies might be taken from other areas that could be affected, such as the bone marrow. You may have more tests and scans to give doctors information about the exact type and stage of the lymphoma you have. All of these investigations help your medical team decide how best to treat you and when to begin treatment.

9.6.1 What other tests might I have?

Fine needle aspiration cytology

Occasionally, a fine needle aspiration cytology (FNAC or FNA) is done if lymphoma is suspected. Small amounts of tissue are collected from a lymph node using a very fine needle.

FNA involves a thin needle being put into a lymph node for 30–40 seconds. A small amount of material is then extracted and sent to a histopathologist. For lymph nodes under the skin, the procedure is done without an anaesthetic. For deeper lymph nodes, or where FNA is done with ultrasound or CT guidance, it is done under a local anaesthetic.

FNA may tell doctors whether there is a possibility that lymphoma is present. However, it is not enough on its own; further tests (such as excision biopsy) are needed to confirm the diagnosis.

FNA is a very safe procedure. In most cases, you can go home immediately afterwards.

Endobronchial ultrasound-guided fine needle aspiration

You may have endobronchial ultrasound-guided fine needle aspiration (EBUS-FNA) if the affected lymph nodes are deep within your chest and are difficult to biopsy.

The procedure involves passing a flexible tube down your windpipe. The tube contains a needle and an instrument called an 'ultrasound probe'. Ultrasound guides the needle to the lymph nodes within the chest. Tissue is collected using the needle.

EBUS-FNA is done while you are under local anaesthetic, with sedation and pain relief. It takes about 30 minutes and you can go home about 2–3 hours after the procedure.

9.7 Here are the answers to some frequently asked questions and concerns about biopsies.

9.7.1 Is a biopsy painful?

A biopsy is done under anaesthetic so it painless. Once the anaesthetic wears off, you might feel some discomfort, such as soreness or aching in the biopsied area. Usually, you are advised to take paracetamol or ibuprofen to relieve any pain. Your doctor or nurse might give you some other painkillers. Any pain should go away completely after a few days.

9.7.2 Can removing a lymph node affect my immunity?

Lymph nodes are an important part of your immune system. The human body has a network of several hundred lymph nodes; removing a small number does not affect your immunity.

9.7.3 Does removing an affected lymph node remove the lymphoma?

A lymph node biopsy tells whether or not lymphoma is present and what type of lymphoma it is. However, the procedure does not remove the lymphoma completely, even if the lymphoma is mostly in one area. Even for lymphomas that appear to be in one area only, surgery usually leaves some cells behind. For this reason, treatments such as chemotherapy and radiotherapy are much more effective.

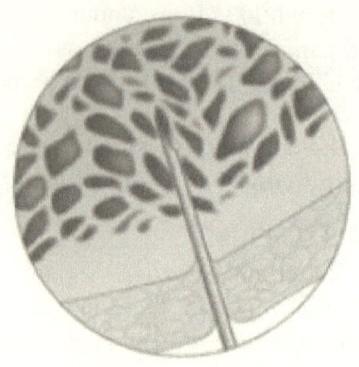

9.8 Bone marrow tests

These test whether lymphoma is in your bone marrow, which is where blood cells are made.

10 Bone marrow biopsy

This page is about bone marrow biopsy, a test you might have to check if you have lymphoma in your bone marrow.

10.1 What is bone marrow?

Bone marrow is the spongy tissue in the centre of some of our bigger bones, such as the thigh bones, the breastbone, pelvis and back bones. The bone marrow is where blood cells are made. It contains basic cells called 'blood stem cells' that can develop into more specialised blood cells, such as white blood cells, red blood cells and platelets. The different types of blood cells are then released into the bloodstream.

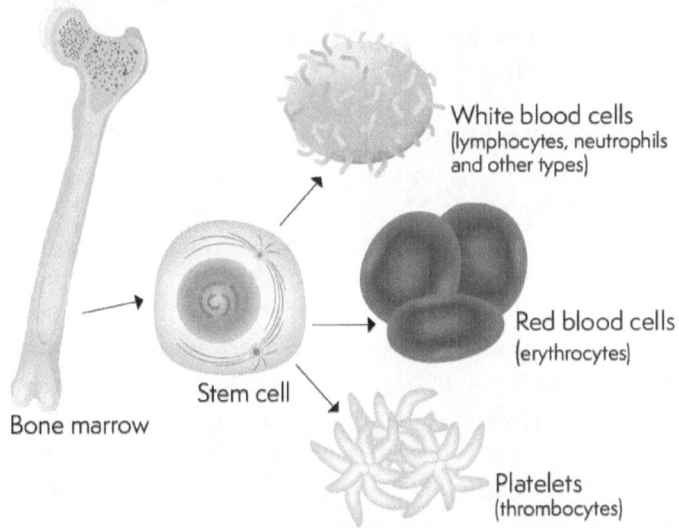

Figure: The different blood cells that develop in the bone marrow

10.2 What is a bone marrow biopsy?

A bone marrow biopsy (also called a 'bone marrow test') is a test where samples of bone marrow are taken.

Two types of bone marrow sample are usually taken:

- **bone marrow aspirate,** which takes a little of the liquid found in the bone marrow space
- **bone marrow trephine,** which takes a small sample of harder bone marrow tissue.

The samples are examined under a microscope to see if any lymphoma cells are present. Other tests may also be done on your bone marrow samples.

10.3 Who might need a bone marrow biopsy?

Bone marrow biopsy might be done for people with many types of lymphoma. It's usually only done if your doctor suspects that lymphoma might be in your bone marrow. This test is then part of 'staging' of the lymphoma – finding out how far it has spread and how it is affecting you. If lymphoma cells are in your bone marrow, it might affect what treatment you need.

A bone marrow biopsy might also be done as part of diagnosing some types of lymphoma that often affect the bone marrow or blood.

If lymphoma is found in your bone marrow, you might need another bone marrow biopsy in the future to check your response to treatment.

Not everyone with lymphoma needs a bone marrow biopsy. Your doctor decides what tests you need based on your individual circumstances.

10.4 What is the process for having a bone marrow biopsy?

Most people who need a bone marrow biopsy have the procedure as an outpatient and do not have to stay in hospital overnight.

10.4.1 How should I prepare?

You should be given information about the procedure and how to prepare for it. You might have blood tests before your procedure to check that your blood clots normally.

Tell your medical team about any medicines, vitamins and other supplements you are taking, or if you have had any reactions to anaesthetics before. If you are taking medicine to thin your blood, you may be asked to stop this before the procedure.

If you feel very anxious, or you found a previous biopsy painful, you might be able to have a sedative to help you relax for the procedure. Sedatives are only available in certain circumstances and in certain centres. They are not recommended for everyone. Some units give 'gas and air' (oxygen and nitrous oxide) during the procedure instead of a sedative. Gas and air gives short-acting pain relief that you breathe in yourself when you need it. Discuss the options with your medical team when the test is being planned.

If you are not having sedation, you can eat and drink as normal before the test. If you are having sedation, your medical team can advise you if you need to stop eating or drinking for a time before the test.

10.4.2 What happens during the procedure?

Bone marrow biopsies are usually taken from your pelvis (hip bone). You are usually asked to lie on your side and curl up, with your knees pulled up towards your chest. Rarely, the sample is taken from the sternum (breastbone). In this case, you lie on your back. Make sure you are comfortable when you are in the correct position – you need to keep as still as possible during the procedure.

The doctor cleans the area then injects a local anaesthetic to numb it. When the area is numb, the doctor inserts a special needle into the space in the middle of the bone and takes a sample of the bone marrow fluid. A second needle is used to take a sample of the harder bone marrow tissue.

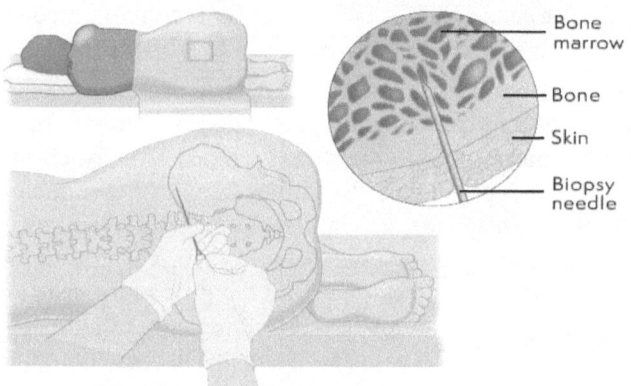

Figure: Bone marrow biopsy

The needle is removed when the sample has been collected. The doctor or nurse puts a dressing over the area where the needles were inserted.

The whole procedure usually takes 10–15 minutes.

Having a bone marrow test can be uncomfortable but any pain or discomfort is usually brief.

- The local anaesthetic can sting or hurt for a few seconds as it goes in, but the site (area) then goes numb.

- When the liquid is taken there can be a pulling feeling or a sharp pain but this should pass almost immediately.
- When the sample of harder tissue is taken, you might feel a dull ache and a pushing sensation or a feeling of pressure building up, but this also passes quickly.

10.4.3 What happens after the procedure?

You need to stay lying down for 15–30 minutes after the procedure to be monitored to make sure there is no bleeding. You might then be asked to rest in the waiting room and have a drink before you go home.

If you have had a sedative, you will be drowsy for a few hours afterwards. You should not drive home or travel on your own – bring someone with you who can take you home. Do not drive or operate machinery for the rest of the day.

The local anaesthetic wears off after 2–3 hours and the area where the needle was inserted can be sore. If you are uncomfortable, take pain relief such as paracetamol regularly over the next few days. Ask your medical team for advice if you need stronger pain relief or if the pain continues for more than a few days.

You can usually return to your normal activities once any pain has settled down.

Keep your dressing on for at least 24 hours or until any bleeding has stopped. Do not get the dressing or sample site wet during this time.

10.5 Is a bone marrow biopsy safe?

A bone marrow biopsy is usually a very safe procedure. Some people have pain after the procedure, but this is usually easily treated with pain relief and gets better within a few days. Seek advice from your medical team if problems persist or are severe.

Serious complications are rare but could include infection or bleeding from the area where the sample was taken.

The area is monitored after the procedure but it can start to bleed again after you go home. If this happens, press down on the area with a dressing until it stops. Contact your medical team if the bleeding doesn't stop when you apply pressure.

Infection is rare but contact your medical team if you develop **any** of the following:

- fever (temperature above 38°C)
- increased pain at the sample site
- redness or swelling at the sample site.

It can be difficult for you to see the sample site so you might need to ask a relative or friend to check for any signs of bleeding or redness.

Your medical team should give you further information on what to look for and when to seek advice.

10.6 When will I get the results?

It can take anywhere from a couple of days to a couple of weeks to get the results of your bone marrow biopsy, depending what tests are done on the sample. Usually, your doctor discusses the results with you at your next appointment. Waiting for test results can make you feel anxious but your medical team are gathering important information during this time so that they can give you the best possible treatment.

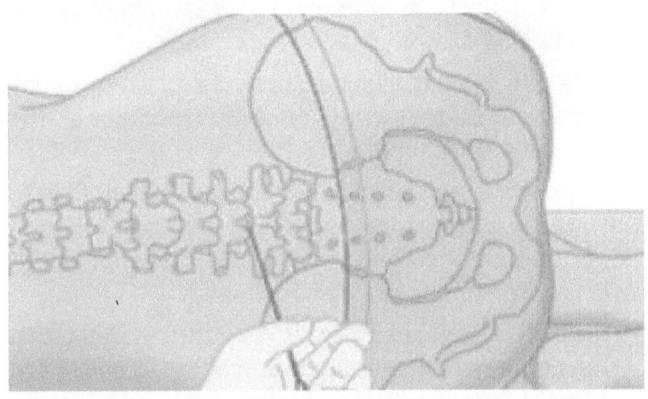

10.7 Lumbar puncture

This test shows if lymphoma is in your central nervous system.

11 Lumbar puncture

A lumbar puncture tests a sample of fluid from your spine. You might need a lumbar puncture if your doctor suspects your lymphoma might be in your central nervous system (CNS; brain and spinal cord) or to give you chemotherapy that reaches your CNS.

11.1 What is a lumbar puncture?

A lumbar puncture (also called a 'spinal tap') is a test that can be used to check for lymphoma cells in the cerebrospinal fluid (CSF). This fluid protects and cushions your brain and spinal cord.

The sample of CSF is examined under a microscope to see if any lymphoma cells are present. Other tests may also be done on your CSF sample.

The results of a lumbar puncture help doctors to decide if you need treatment that reaches your central nervous system (CNS; brain and spinal cord).

A lumbar puncture may also be done to give chemotherapy directly into the CSF so that it can reach the CNS. This way of giving treatment is called 'intrathecal chemotherapy'. You might have intrathecal chemotherapy:

- as a preventive treatment if your doctors think there is a high risk of lymphoma spreading to your CNS. This is known as 'CNS prophylaxis'
- to treat lymphoma of the brain, spinal cord or eye (CNS lymphoma).

11.2 Who might need a lumbar puncture?

Lymphoma cells are sometimes found in the CSF in some types of high-grade non-Hodgkin lymphoma, for example:

- Burkitt lymphoma
- diffuse large B-cell lymphoma (DLBCL)
- T-cell lymphoma
- CNS lymphoma.

Not everyone with these types of lymphoma needs a lumbar puncture. Your doctor decides what tests you need based on your individual circumstances.

11.3 What is the process for having a lumbar puncture?

Most people who need a lumbar puncture have the procedure as an outpatient and do not have to stay in hospital overnight.

11.3.1 How should I prepare?

You should be given information about the procedure and how to prepare for it. You may have a blood test before the procedure to check that you don't have any problems with blood clotting. You can eat and drink as normal before the test. Tell your medical team about any medicines, vitamins and other supplements you are taking. If you are taking medicine to thin your blood, you may be asked to stop this before the procedure.

11.3.2 What happens during the procedure?

Your details, such as your name and date of birth, are checked before the procedure.

You are usually asked to lie on your side and curl up, with your knees pulled up towards your chest. Sometimes, it is easier for you and your doctor if the test is done while you are sitting up instead. In this case, you are asked to sit leaning forwards onto a pillow that is resting on a table in front of you. Make sure you are comfortable – you need to keep as still as possible during the procedure.

When you are in the correct position, the doctor feels for a gap between your vertebrae (bones of your spine) in your lower back. The doctor cleans the area then injects a local anaesthetic. A few people, particularly children, might be given a sedative to help them relax. When the area is numb, the doctor inserts a special needle into the space containing CSF.

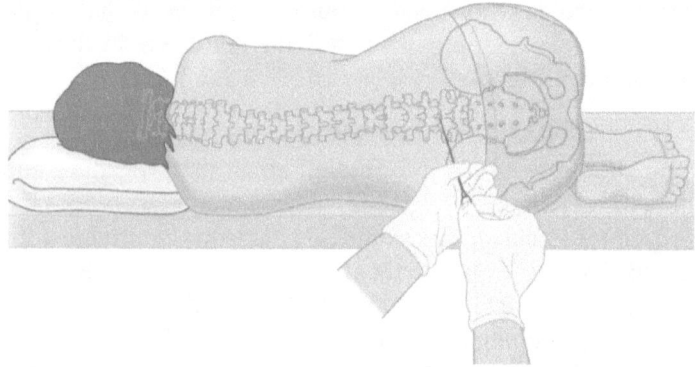

Figure: Lumbar puncture needle going into the lower spine

When the needle is in the right place, CSF starts to drip out. The doctor collects a small amount of the fluid (usually around one teaspoon or 5 ml). It only takes a few seconds. This test isn't usually painful but it might be uncomfortable and the local anaesthetic can sting.

If you are having intrathecal chemotherapy, the drugs are injected through the needle. You might have samples of CSF taken and intrathecal chemotherapy given during the same procedure if needed.

The needle is then removed. The doctor or nurse puts a plaster or dressing over the tiny hole left by the needle. You can remove this the next day.

11.3.3 What happens after the procedure?

You might be asked to lie down flat for a while after the procedure. This may reduce the risk of developing a headache. Drinking plenty, including caffeinated drinks like tea, coffee and coke, might also help. Although there is no clear evidence that these measures reduce the risk of a headache, many haematology teams recommend them. Most people can go home the same day.

Headaches are very common after a lumbar puncture. A headache can develop several hours or the day after the procedure and can last for several days. If you develop a headache after going home, you should lie down and rest until it eases. Make sure you have pain relief medication available in case you need them. Ask your medical team for advice on which pain relief medications are best before you go home.

11.4 Is a lumbar puncture safe?

A lumbar puncture is usually a very safe procedure. The main risks are developing headaches, or pain and swelling at the injection site. These problems generally get better on their own. Seek advice from your medical team if problems persist or are severe. Serious complications are very rare but could include infection or bleeding. Contact your medical team if you develop any of the following:

- fever (temperature above 38°C)
- sensitivity to bright lights
- vomiting (being sick)
- blood or fluid around the injection site
- tingling or numbness in your legs.

11.5 When will I get the results?

It can take anywhere from a couple of days to a couple of weeks to get the results of your lumbar puncture, depending what tests are done on the sample. Waiting for test results can be an anxious time but your medical team are gathering important information at this time so they can give you the best possible treatment.

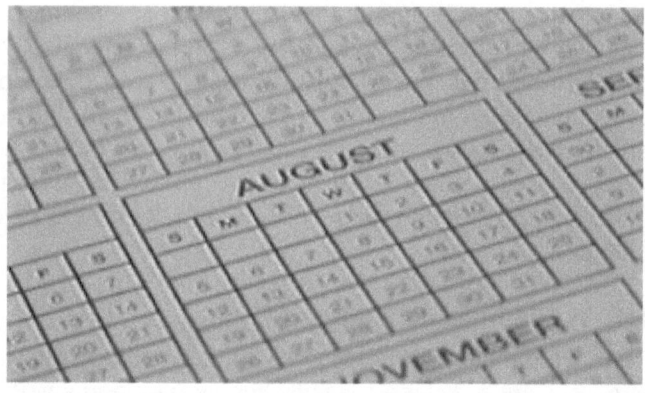

11.6 Waiting for your results

How long do I need to wait for my test results?

The time you wait for your test results can vary greatly.

Sometimes, results are available very quickly, within a couple of days. This is usually if the results are clear and the tests have been analysed urgently. The waiting time also depends on the type of test you had. Blood test results are usually available quickly. It takes longer for samples to be prepared and experts to be available to look at other tests like biopsy samples and scans.

In most cases, it takes a couple of weeks to get test results. It can take longer to get the results of tests that are not urgent, for example, tests that are part of your routine follow-up. More specialist tests can also take longer. For example, if the samples need to be sent to another laboratory or expert.

Do not be alarmed if it takes longer than usual to get the results of tests. It does not mean something is wrong – there are many possible reasons for a delay.

You might be given an initial diagnosis then have more tests to find out more about the lymphoma. This helps your medical team recommend the best treatment for you.

Your medical team should be able to give you an idea of how long your test results will take. Talk to them if you are unsure or if your results are taking longer than you expected.

Why do I need to wait for my test results?
The wait for test results might seem long. However, there is a lot going on between the time you have your test and the time you get the results. The person doing the test is not usually trained to interpret the information they collect. The information is passed on to a specialist.

If you had an X-ray or a scan, a radiologist examines the images.

Blood samples are tested in a laboratory.

The samples, for example, from a biopsy, bone marrow tests or lumbar puncture, are prepared in a specialised laboratory and examined by expert pathologists. The samples may need to be sent from your local hospital to the specialised laboratory.

Some samples take longer to prepare than others; for example, the tissue in bone marrow tests has to be decalcified (calcium removed) before the sample can be examined.

The specialists write a report about your test results. Reports are sent to the doctor who ordered the test, usually your consultant. In most cases, your doctor waits until they have reviewed the information from all of your tests before they contact you. Your doctor does not want to risk giving you an incorrect diagnosis or treatment that is not suitable for you. Several different people with different specialities need to look at your tests and discuss your results. This group of people is known as a 'multidisciplinary team' (MDT). If you have a rare type of lymphoma, there might be more people involved in making sure you have the correct diagnosis and the best care.

When all the information is available, your doctor arranges an appointment with you to discuss the results of the tests.

There are many possible reasons for test results to take longer than expected, for example:

More specialised tests might be needed on samples. For example, cells from a biopsy are looked at under a microscope using different stains (dyes). This is usually enough to make a diagnosis but other tests might be needed to look at the cells in more detail.

Samples may need to be sent away to a different laboratory if specialised tests are needed, for example to look at the proteins in a tissue sample.

The specialist might need a second opinion. Samples and images might need to be sent to an expert at another hospital, particularly for rare types of lymphoma.

The results of one test might mean that your doctor recommends further tests. For example, if a scan identifies a possible problem, you might need a biopsy or a different type of scan to look at an area in more detail.

A test might need to be repeated, for example, if there were not enough cells in the sample collected.

It is very important that your medical team know exactly what type of lymphoma you have and how it is affecting you. This information helps them plan the best treatment for you.

A delay of a couple of weeks while waiting for test results is very unlikely to affect your outcome. Your doctor can request that your test results are prioritised if they are needed urgently.

How can I cope emotionally while waiting for test results?

Waiting for test results can bring a great deal of uncertainty and give rise to some difficult emotional responses. You might start to imagine the worst possible scenario or have a general sense of anxiety or fear.

While these emotions are natural and may not go away entirely, there are some simple things you could do to help manage them.

Write down your worries

Often, worries go round in our head, which can be exhausting. Try to 'catch' these thoughts before they spiral out of control. Simply getting your thoughts down on paper can take away some of their power and bring a sense of release. Seeing your worries in writing may also help you to identify any links between them and help you to consider how to address them.

If you find that worries start to take over your thoughts, try setting aside 'worry time' – contained time to think about your worries. Write down any worries or concerns as they come into your mind. Keep a notepad by your bed in case they come into your mind during the night. Tell yourself that you will return to your worries and give them your full attention later.

Identify strategies

Try to pin-point what underlies your worry and then think about how you can help yourself.

For example:

Worry

'If I'm given a diagnosis of lymphoma, I won't know how to deal with it. I know nothing about lymphoma or what it could mean for me.'

Strategies

Reconsider unhelpful thoughts, for example: 'I don't have a diagnosis now so I will take one day at a time. If I am diagnosed with lymphoma, I will have an opportunity to ask questions and to find out my options'.

Useful resources

Medical professionals who give you your test results can answer your questions and give you more information about lymphoma and your treatment options.

Lymphoma Action offers information about lymphoma and emotional support to people affected by lymphoma.

Worry

'I feel totally overwhelmed. I can't deal with the uncertainty'.

Strategies

Make time for yourself (for example, take a walk, spend time with friends or have a relaxing bath).

Try stress relieving techniques (breathing exercises, meditation or mindfulness).

Talk to someone close to you about how you feel.

Focus your energies on something creative, for example paint or sing.

Useful resources

Your doctors can discuss your anxieties with you. They may also be able to refer you for specialist psychological support with your emotions.

Lymphoma Action's support services. For example, you may find it helps to talk to others who can relate to your situation through online forums and support groups.

I found that waiting for test results and fearing the unknown made for a stressful time. Remember that you are not alone. Online forums can be a great source of support to read or 'chat' about experiences.

Where can I find support?

Going for tests and scans for lymphoma will have an emotional impact. However, if your level of distress continues or worsens and affects your everyday life, you may find it beneficial to seek additional support.

This could include a talking therapy, such as counselling or another type of psychological support. Ask your doctor if they can refer you on the NHS, or search for a private practitioner online. You can search for a private therapist in your area on the British Association for Counselling and Psychotherapy website. You can also use the British Psychological Society's search tool.

Everyone finds their own way, so do what's right for you. I found that positive distractions really helped me. I listened to music, went out with friends, baked, read or tried something new – anything to keep my mind occupied. I would suggest using the internet with caution. Don't let it fuel your anxieties.

K, diagnosed with Hodgkin lymphoma

Remember that your medical team is there to support you. This includes listening to any concerns you have, answering your questions and suggesting ways to help you. You can find self-help strategies and support with coping with challenging feelings online through various websites, including the Mental Health Foundation, Mind, and Moodjuice.

You may also find our Living with lymphoma booklet helpful. It describes some of the feelings and emotions you may have if you have been diagnosed with lymphoma and suggests ways to help you manage these.

Find out more about how the Lymphoma Action can support you.

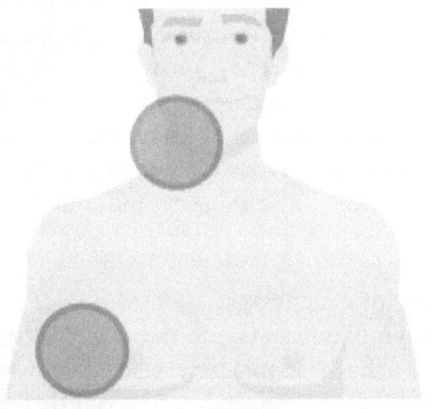

11.7 Stages of lymphoma

Staging of lymphoma

Staging of Hodgkin and non-Hodgkin lymphoma in adults. Staging is also called 'grouping' or 'classifying'. Different staging systems are used for B-cell skin lymphoma and T-cell skin lymphoma, as well as non-Hodgkin lymphoma in children.

What is staging?

Stages of lymphoma

'Early' stage and 'advanced' stage

Lymphoma grade

What is staging and why is it done?

'Staging' is the process of working out which parts of your body contain lymphoma. The tests and scans you have when you are diagnosed help the doctors to work out the stage.

Doctors group lymphomas into different stages because it helps them to plan treatment. They know from many years of research that particular stages respond best to particular amounts, types and combinations of treatments. Generally, staging is the same for most types of lymphoma. The same staging system is used for Hodgkin and non-Hodgkin lymphomas in adults.

There are a couple of exceptions:
Cutaneous (skin) lymphomas start in the skin (rather than having spread there from somewhere else). They behave differently to other lymphomas and are staged differently, too.

Staging for non-Hodgkin lymphoma in children is also slightly different to staging in adults.

What are the stages of lymphoma?
Staging in adults is the same for Hodgkin and non-Hodgkin lymphoma. There are 4 main stages of lymphoma. These are numbered 1 to 4, sometimes written in Roman numerals as I to IV. Letters after the numbers can also appear.

Stage 1

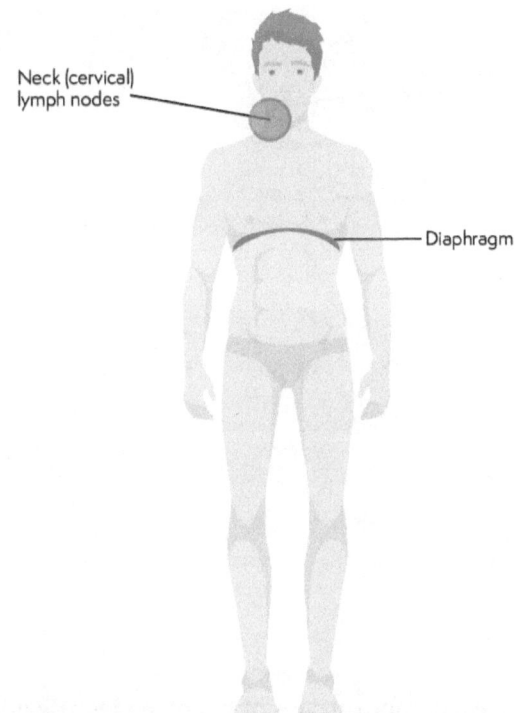

Stage 1: One group of lymph nodes affected either above or below the diaphragm

Stage 1 means that there is lymphoma in only 1 group of lymph nodes (glands). The diagram shows these in the neck, but they can be anywhere in the body, either above or below the diaphragm.

Stage 1E lymphoma means that the lymphoma started in a single body organ outside the lymphatic system and is only in that organ. This is called extranodal lymphoma.

Stage 2

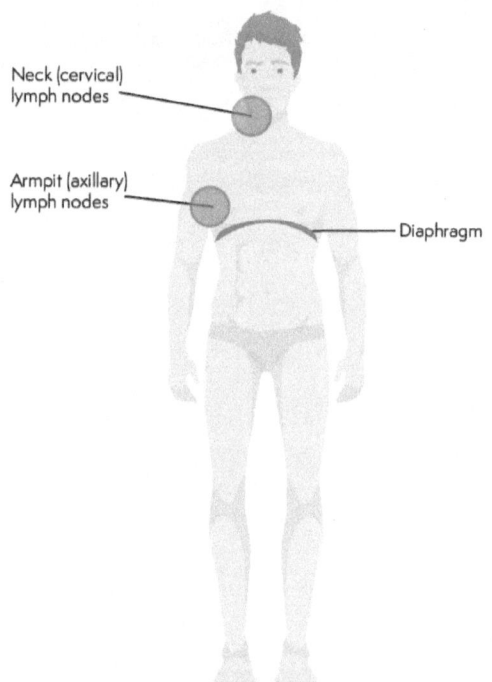

Stage 2: Two or more groups of lymph nodes affected either above or below the diaphragm

Stage 2 means that there is lymphoma in 2 or more groups of lymph nodes. These can be anywhere in the body, but to be diagnosed with stage 2 lymphoma, they must all be on the same side of the diaphragm.

In extranodal lymphoma, stage 2E means there is lymphoma that started in 1 body organ and is also in 1 or more groups of lymph nodes. These must all be on the same side of the diaphragm.

You may see a number in a smaller font next to the stage, for example stage 2₃. This 'smaller' number tells you how many groups of lymph nodes contain lymphoma. On the diagram, this is stage 2 lymphoma, with lymphoma cells in 3 groups of lymph nodes.

Stage 3

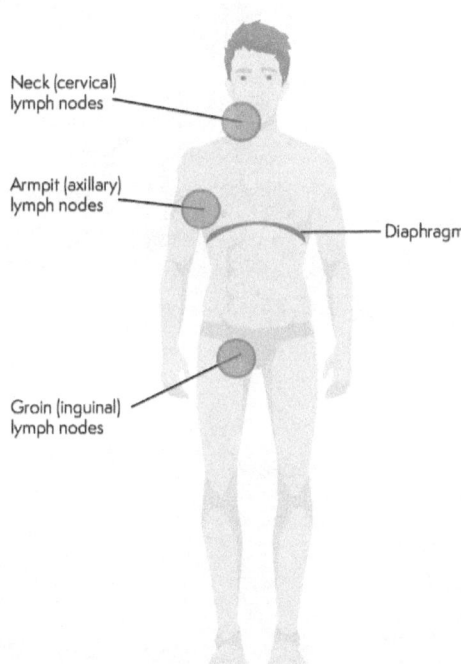

Stage 3: Lymph nodes affected on both sides of the diaphragm

Stage 3 means that there are lymph nodes that contain lymphoma on both sides of the diaphragm.

Stage 4

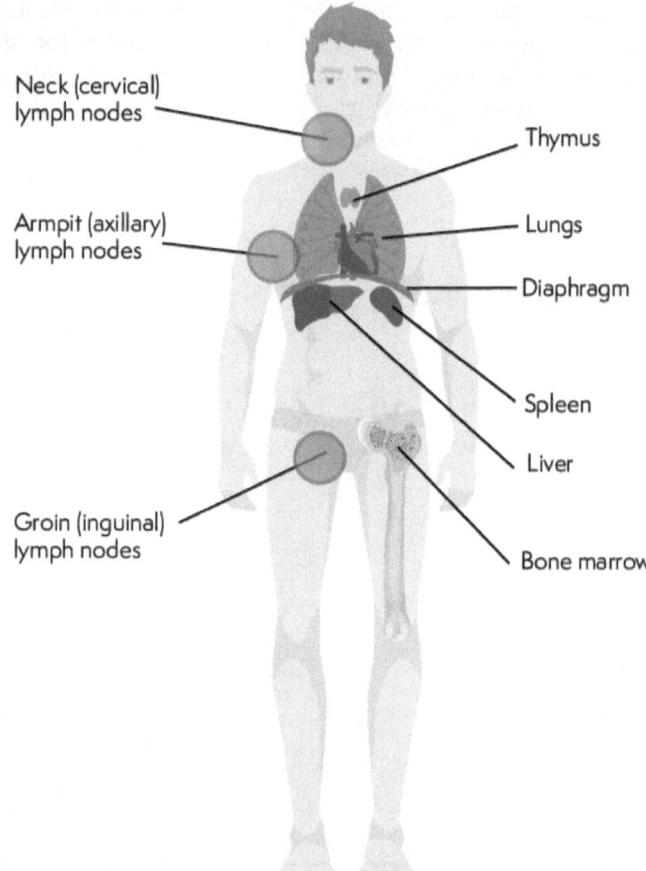

Stage 4: Lymphoma is found either in organs outside the lymphatic system or in the bone marrow

Stage 4 is the most advanced stage of lymphoma. Lymphoma cells have spread to at least 1 body organ outside the lymphatic system, for example, the lungs, liver, bone marrow or solid bones.

The spleen and the thymus are part of the lymphatic system, so lymphoma in those organs only does not count as stage 4.

Letters after your stage

You may have 'A' or 'B' after your number stage. 'A' means you don't have any of a set of general symptoms. 'B' means you have 1 or more of these general symptoms:

unintentional weight loss (more than 10% in the 6 months before you were diagnosed)

night sweats

fevers (temperatures above 38°C).

Doctors sometimes call these 'B symptoms'.

For example, if your stage is 2A, you have lymphoma in 2 or more groups of lymph nodes on the same side of your diaphragm and you haven't had any of the B symptoms.

If your lymphoma is stage 1B, you have lymphoma in 1 group of lymph nodes and you have had at least 1 of the B symptoms.

Extranodal lymphoma and lymphoma in the spleen

Doctors also sometimes use the letter 'E', which stands for 'extranodal'. It means that the lymphoma started in a body organ that is not part of the lymphatic system, for example, in the digestive system or in the salivary glands. It doesn't include lymphoma that has spread to a body organ.

The spleen and the thymus are body organs that are part of the lymphatic system. Lymphoma that is in these organs is not regarded as extranodal. If you have lymphoma in the spleen, your doctor may put 'S' after your stage; 1S is stage 1 lymphoma that is only in the spleen.

What do 'early' stage and 'advanced' stage mean?

You may hear your doctor talk about 'early' stage or 'advanced' stage lymphoma. This is a simplified version of the staging described above.

'Early' stage means that you have either stage 1 or stage 2 lymphoma. The lymph nodes that contain lymphoma cells are all on the same side of your diaphragm.

'Advanced' stage means that you have either stage 3 or stage 4 lymphoma. The lymph nodes containing lymphoma cells are on both sides of your diaphragm, or there is lymphoma that has spread to body organs outside your lymphatic system, such as your bone marrow, liver or lungs.

The lymphatic system is all over the body, so it isn't unusual to find that lymphoma is widespread when it is diagnosed. Unlike many other cancers, stage 4 lymphoma can be successfully treated. Depending on the exact type of lymphoma, it may be cured or kept under control for a long time. It is important for doctors to stage your lymphoma accurately. Correctly identifying the stage of your lymphoma helps them to decide on the most suitable treatment, and gives them a baseline to monitor how well treatment is working.

What does 'grade' mean?
You may hear your doctor talk about the 'grade' of your lymphoma. The grade describes what the lymphoma cells look like under a microscope.

The grade of your lymphoma also helps your doctor to decide which treatment is best for you.

Non-Hodgkin lymphoma is usually classed as either 'high-grade' or 'low-grade'. High-grade lymphoma means that the cells look like they are dividing quite quickly. This means the lymphoma is likely to be relatively fast-growing.

In low-grade lymphoma the cells look like they are dividing more slowly. This means the lymphoma is slower to develop. Follicular lymphoma is the most common type of low-grade lymphoma.

Grading of follicular lymphoma
People with follicular lymphoma might also be given a numbered grade: 1, 2 or 3. This relates to the number of large, follicular lymphoma cells (centroblasts) that can be seen under a microscope:

Grade 1 means that there are between 0 and 5 large cells.

Grade 2 means that there are between 6 and 15 large cells.

Grade 3 means that there are more than 15 large cells.

Grade 3 can be divided into 3A and 3B. In 3A, there are more than 15 centroblasts. In 3B, the tissue is almost entirely made up of these large lymphoma cells.

Grade makes no real difference to your treatment or likely outcome of follicular lymphoma, apart from 3B, which is regarded as faster growing than the other grades of follicular lymphoma. Grade 3B follicular lymphoma usually behaves and is treated like diffuse large B-cell lymphoma, which is a high-grade lymphoma.

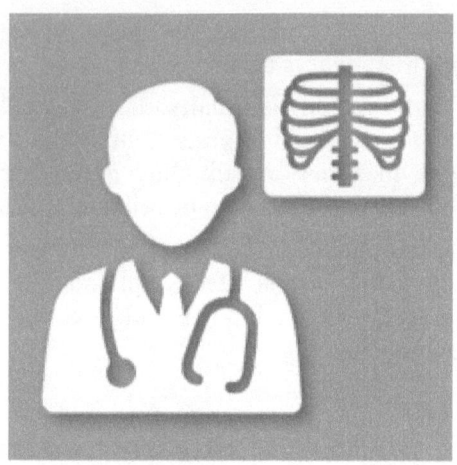

12 Treatment for lymphoma

Different lymphomas may need different treatment. Your general health and the stage of your lymphoma are also important in deciding what treatment is best for you. This page gives you a brief overview of treatment for lymphoma and tells you where to find more information.

12.1 How do my medical team decide what treatment I need?

Your treatment is planned individually. It is planned and managed by a team of health professionals who are specialists in different areas. Together, they are known as a multidisciplinary team. One specialist is responsible for your overall care.

Your medical team aim to offer you treatment that has the best chance of successfully treating your lymphoma with the least damage to your long-term health.

There are guidelines for the treatment of many types of lymphoma. For example, the British Society for Haematology produces guidelines for haematologists. However, your medical team considers several factors when deciding on the best treatment for you.

Lymphoma-specific factors, like:

- the type of lymphoma you have
- the stage of your disease
- the size of any lumps of lymphoma
- what parts of your body are affected by lymphoma
- your symptoms
- results of genetic tests on your lymphoma, which can tell the doctor if you are likely to respond to certain treatments.

Individual factors, like:

- your age and future plans, eg if you are of childbearing age your doctor might suggest treatment that is less likely to reduce your fertility
- your general health
- any other medical conditions you have
- any other medication you need.

Children and young people under 18 are often given different treatment to adults. If you are under 18 or are the parent or carer of a child with lymphoma, you might want to read our section dedicated to children and young people.

12.2 What do I need to know about my treatment?

Your medical team should talk to you about your treatment before it starts. They should explain:

- the aim of your treatment – whether it aims to cure or control your lymphoma
- the exact drugs they want to use
- how often you are to be given treatment and how long it normally takes
- how your treatment is given
- how often you need to attend the hospital and whether you need to stay overnight
- any side effects you might develop, including late effects (side effects that develop months or years after treatment)
- what to look out for and where to get help if you have any problems during your treatment.

12.3 Where can I find more information about treatment for lymphoma?

Our information on types of lymphoma outlines the treatment most commonly used for each type of lymphoma. Your specialist might recommend a different treatment to those most commonly used depending on your individual circumstances.

You can find out more about how your type of treatment is given on our dedicated pages, including:

- chemotherapy
- radiotherapy
- antibody therapy, including rituximab
- steroids
- stem cell transplants
- targeted drugs.

Macmillan also produces useful information about treatment for cancer, including information on different chemotherapy drugs and regimens (combinations of drugs).

Your specialist might ask you to consider being treated as part of a clinical trial (a scientific study that tests medical treatments).

Treatment is only part of your care when you have lymphoma. You might also find our information on living with lymphoma useful. It includes ways to support your body through your treatment and recovery, information on your emotional wellbeing and advice on dealing with the day-to-day practicalities of life with lymphoma.

13 Active monitoring (watch and wait)

Sometimes, lymphoma doesn't need treatment straightaway. This information page is about active monitoring – where your lymphoma is monitored until you need treatment. Active monitoring is also called 'watch and wait' or sometimes 'active surveillance'.

13.1 What is active monitoring?

Some types of lymphoma grow slowly and may not cause any problems, at least for a while. If this is the case for you, your doctor might suggest active monitoring of the lymphoma.

Active monitoring (sometimes called 'active surveillance') is where you have regular check-ups with your medical team to monitor your health and to see how the lymphoma is affecting you. You do not have any treatment for the lymphoma until it is causing significant health problems.

You might hear this approach called 'watch and wait':

- 'watch' because you have regular check-ups (monitoring)
- 'wait' because you wait until the lymphoma is causing troublesome problems before you have treatment.

You might have active monitoring when you are diagnosed or after a course of treatment that has left some lymphoma behind.

13.2 Why is active monitoring done?

It can be difficult to understand why your doctor is suggesting you do not have any treatment for your cancer.

Low-grade (slow-growing) types of lymphoma often respond well to treatment, but are usually difficult to cure (get rid of permanently). People with low-grade lymphoma often live for many years and have courses of treatment from time-to-time.

On average, people who are not having troublesome problems from their lymphoma live just as long if they save treatment until it is needed rather than having treatment straightaway. If you have mild symptoms that you can cope with, it might still be better to reserve treatment until the lymphoma is causing problems that are harder to manage.

Some people never need treatment for low-grade lymphoma or do not need treatment for many years. Active monitoring saves them unnecessary treatment.

There can be advantages to having active monitoring instead of immediate treatment:

- there is no risk of side effects or late effects from treatment
- the lymphoma cells won't become resistant (do not respond) to treatment

- fewer hospital visits - you only need to go to appointments for outpatient check-ups
- most people enjoy a good quality of life and respond just as well to treatment when it is really needed.

Active monitoring does **not** mean that:
- there is no treatment available for your lymphoma
- you are too old to be treated, or that
- your doctors are trying to save money on your treatment.

As it is difficult to get rid of low-grade lymphoma completely, there is often some lymphoma left after treatment. If the leftover lymphoma is not causing problems, you are likely to have active monitoring again after treatment.

13.3 Who might have active monitoring?

Types of low-grade non-Hodgkin lymphoma that might be monitored after diagnosis or between treatment courses include:

- follicular lymphoma
- marginal zone lymphomas (MALT lymphoma, splenic marginal zone lymphoma or nodal marginal zone lymphoma)
- Waldenström's macroglobulinaemia (lymphoplasmacytic lymphoma)
- chronic lymphocytic leukaemia (CLL) / small lymphocytic lymphoma (SLL).

Mantle cell lymphoma is usually fast-growing, but some people have an 'indolent' form of mantle cell lymphoma that grows much more slowly than usual. If you have indolent mantle cell lymphoma, you might not need treatment straightaway. Most people do need treatment at some time.

Some people with nodular lymphocyte-predominant Hodgkin lymphoma (NLPHL) also have active monitoring after the affected lymph nodes have been removed. NLPHL is an uncommon and usually slow-growing type of Hodgkin lymphoma.

Active monitoring is only suggested if you have a slow-growing type of lymphoma and:

- you are well
- you have no troublesome symptoms from your lymphoma
- you have small lymph nodes that are not causing problems and are not growing rapidly
- your blood tests don't detect any significant problems
- none of your major organs (for example, heart, lungs, kidneys) are being affected by the lymphoma.

You can watch personal experience videos of people on active monitoring for different types of lymphoma on our active monitoring playlist.

13.3.1 Are there any other options?

Your medical team should discuss all the treatment options with you.

Some people with follicular lymphoma and no troublesome symptoms have a short course of an antibody treatment, for example, rituximab, before going on to active monitoring. Rituximab is given once a week for 4 weeks. Recent evidence suggests this approach does not extend the time you might live but could delay the time until you need stronger treatment. This delay could mean that more people never need stronger treatment.

13.4 What happens on active monitoring?

If you are on active monitoring, you have regular check-ups with your doctor, clinical nurse specialist or another member of your medical team to make sure your lymphoma doesn't need treatment.

They talk to you about how you're feeling and whether you've noticed any change in your symptoms or any new symptoms. They will also examine you. This might include:

- taking your temperature, pulse, blood pressure and weight
- listening to your heart and lungs
- feeling your abdomen (tummy), armpits, groin and neck to check for enlarged lymph nodes or other signs that your lymphoma may need treatment.

You also have blood tests to check your blood count, look for signs of inflammation or infection, and make sure your bone marrow, liver and kidneys are working as they should be.

Depending on the type of lymphoma you have, where it is in your body and the results of your examination and blood tests, you might also need further tests such as a CT scan or PET scan.

Your follow-up appointments are usually every couple of months for the first year, then every 3–6 months if your lymphoma hasn't got worse.

If you notice any change in your symptoms or any new symptoms, don't wait for your next appointment – contact your medical team straight away. They can reassure you or see you sooner if necessary. Remember that you are on active monitoring because you have a slow-growing type of lymphoma, so urgent treatment is rarely needed even if you start to develop symptoms.

13.5 When does treatment start?

The time until treatment is needed varies considerably depending on what type of lymphoma you have and your individual circumstances. You might need treatment soon after diagnosis, or after a treatment course, but you might not need treatment for many years. Some people never need treatment for their lymphoma.

Your medical team are likely to suggest treatment if:

- your symptoms become too troublesome or you develop symptoms known as 'B symptoms' (night sweats, weight loss and fevers)
- your lymph nodes start to grow more quickly or you develop swollen lymph nodes in new places
- your blood tests or other test results show that lymphoma is affecting your major organs or bone marrow.

Note: You can develop swollen lymph nodes for other reasons, for example infections. You might also have other health conditions that could be causing problems. If you develop new symptoms, your medical team might want to keep a close eye on you for a while or run other tests to decide whether the lymphoma is causing problems. It is important to remember that low-grade lymphomas grow slowly and there is rarely an urgent need to start treatment.

The risk that a lymphoma will transform (change) into a faster-growing (high-grade) lymphoma may concern some people with low-grade lymphoma or nodular lymphocyte-predominant Hodgkin lymphoma (NLPHL). Your medical team check for signs of transformation at your appointments, but it is important that you are aware of these signs and find out when and how to seek advice.

Do not wait until your next appointment if you develop new or worsening symptoms or have concerns that your lymphoma might be getting worse. Contact your medical team to discuss your concerns. They can reassure you or might want to arrange an earlier appointment or tests for you.

If your medical team think you need to start treatment, they can explain why and discuss the treatment options with you.

13.6 Living with active monitoring

Some people feel relieved that they don't need treatment yet. Others find it hard at first to know that they have lymphoma but are not having treatment to get rid of it. It can be difficult to believe you don't need treatment and it's not unusual to feel you're being 'fobbed off'. You may feel angry or frustrated and you probably have a lot of questions. These reactions are normal. Your medical team understand what you're going through and should be able to answer any questions you have.

Family and friends might also find it difficult to accept that you don't need treatment. It can be frustrating for you to have to explain it to them – especially if you are struggling to cope with it yourself.

The uncertainty of active monitoring can be very stressful and you may experience ups and downs in your mood. Many people feel anxious in the days or weeks before their check-ups and then feel relieved afterwards. Some people say it's hard to plan for the future because they don't know if or when they'll need treatment.

It's quite common for people on active monitoring to suffer from fatigue. This can be difficult to cope with but there are lots of things you can do to make it easier.

Over time, many people find they get used to being on active monitoring and find a 'new normal' life where they can manage their symptoms. It helps some people to think of their lymphoma as a chronic illness like diabetes or high blood pressure, rather than as a type of cancer.

Talking to your doctor, specialist nurse, a psychologist or one of our Buddies may help. But if you are finding it very hard to cope with being on active monitoring, do make sure you let your medical team know and ask what can be done to help you.

13.6.1 What can I do to help myself?

If you are on active monitoring, it is important that you stay in touch with your medical team and attend your clinic appointments.

There is no evidence to suggest that you can do anything yourself to keep your lymphoma at bay. However, as you might need treatment in future, you might want to prepare for this by getting yourself as healthy as possible. This might mean making changes to your lifestyle, such as:

- eating a healthy diet and trying to maintain a healthy weight
- not smoking

- limiting your alcohol intake
- taking regular exercise.

You might also want to think about your job and responsibilities, particularly if you're struggling with fatigue. By law, your employer must make any 'reasonable adjustments' that allow you to continue working.

Some people on active monitoring like to focus on the things they enjoy doing, such as hobbies, travelling or seeing family and friends. Talk to your medical team about any vaccinations you might need or precautions you should take. Some people struggle to get travel insurance – our forums can offer advice from other people in a similar situation. You might also want to learn more about your lymphoma so that you can make an informed choice when you do need treatment. This helps some people but might make others more anxious, so it's fine if you don't want to do this.

14 Chemotherapy

Chemotherapy is a treatment that uses drugs to kill cancer cells. Chemotherapy can be used alone or in combination with other treatments such as targeted treatments and radiotherapy.

14.1.1 What is the aim of chemotherapy?

Many people with lymphoma have chemotherapy, but not everyone does.

The aim of chemotherapy depends on the exact type of lymphoma you have. Some types of lymphoma can be cured with chemotherapy while others can be effectively controlled with chemotherapy.

14.1.2 How often do I have treatment and how long does a course last?

A course of chemotherapy usually involves several treatments ('cycles'). A rest period follows each cycle. Your doctor decides how many cycles you should have. A whole course of treatment can vary from several weeks to a number of months.

14.1.3 How is chemotherapy given?

Different chemotherapy drugs for lymphoma are given in different ways:

- orally – by mouth
- intravenously (IV) – into a vein
- intrathecally – into the cerebrospinal fluid (CSF), which surrounds the brain and spine.

14.1.4 Is chemotherapy painful?

Having chemotherapy is not painful. There might be times when you feel some discomfort, for example, in your arm if you have intravenous chemotherapy given into a vein in your arm.

14.1.5 What are the side effects of chemotherapy?

Side effects can vary a lot from person-to-person and depend on the exact chemotherapy drugs you are given.

Your medical team should talk to you about the side effects you might have. The following side effects are quite common after chemotherapy; however you are unlikely to have all of them:

- increased risk of infection
- nausea
- hair loss or thinning
- sore mouth and mouth ulcers
- change in taste – foods can taste different, unpleasant or metallic
- fatigue – extreme tiredness
- nail changes – your nails can become brittle and ridged.

Less common side effects depend on the particular type of chemotherapy drug you have.

14.2 What is chemotherapy?

Chemotherapy means treatment with drugs that kill cancer cells. These drugs are known as 'cytotoxic' drugs. 'Cyto' means 'cell' and 'toxic' means 'poison'. Chemotherapy works by 'poisoning' cancerous lymphoma cells.

14.3 How does chemotherapy work?

Lymphoma is a type of cancer. It develops when lymphocytes (specialised white blood cells) grow out of control. They can then build up in the lymph nodes and/or other organs. This can happen when lymphocytes divide more often than normal. It can also happen when they do not die when they should.

Chemotherapy for lymphoma works in one or both of the following ways:

- stopping lymphoma cells from dividing
- triggering lymphoma cells to die.

The drugs work on cells that are in the process of dividing but they have little effect on cells that are not dividing.

Most of our cells have a limited lifespan. They die naturally and new cells replace them. Lymphomas occur when this process goes wrong.

Chemotherapy drugs often work by preventing this process of cell division in the abnormal cells, which leads to the cells dying off.

14.3.1 Chemotherapy regimens (combinations of drugs)

Usually, more than one chemotherapy drug is given at once. This is known as a combination regimen.

Different drugs work on different phases of the cell cycle. Having them together helps to kill as many lymphoma cells as possible.

For some types of lymphoma, chemotherapy drugs are often combined with targeted treatments, such as rituximab. Similarly, steroids are often combined with chemotherapy.

14.4 Why is chemotherapy used to treat lymphoma?

Chemotherapy is often used in the treatment of lymphoma because most lymphoma cells are easily killed by it. Chemotherapy can be used on its own or in combination with other treatments, for example targeted therapy or radiotherapy.

The exact chemotherapy treatment your doctors recommend for you depends on factors including the type and stage of your lymphoma.

14.5 How is chemotherapy given?

You are most likely to have chemotherapy in one or more of the following ways:

- orally (by mouth)
- intravenously (into a vein)
- intrathecally (into the fluid surrounding the brain and spinal cord).

14.5.1 Oral chemotherapy

Oral chemotherapy is taken by mouth, in the form of tablets or capsules. You might have all of your chemotherapy orally.

Oral chemotherapy can be taken safely at home and does not require an overnight hospital stay. You will be given instructions about how to take the tablets at home.

Important: Chemotherapy drugs should not be handled by anyone else other than the person who is taking them.

14.5.2 Intravenous (IV) chemotherapy

Intravenous (IV) chemotherapy means that drugs are given into a vein. This is the most common way to have chemotherapy for lymphoma.

IV chemotherapy can be given:

- through a cannula
- through a central venous catheter ('line').

IV chemotherapy through a cannula

IV chemotherapy for lymphoma is usually given through a cannula, a soft plastic tube with a needle inside it. A nurse or doctor puts the needle into a vein, usually on the back of your hand or in your lower arm. The needle is then removed, leaving only the plastic tube in the vein. You have a dressing put on to keep the cannula clean and in the correct position.

Some IV drugs are given as a 'bolus' or a 'push' dose. The nurse injects the drug through the cannula over a short period of time, usually over a few minutes.

Other drugs are given through an intravenous infusion (drip). IV chemotherapy drugs are mixed with fluid in a bag. The fluid drips slowly from the bag, down some tubing and through a cannula into a vein in your arm over a set amount of time. This could be anywhere from 30 minutes to a number of hours, depending on the drug you are given. Your medical team can advise you how long you will need to be in the chemotherapy unit for this procedure.

The bag must be kept higher than your arm, so it is often hung from a metal drip stand. The stand usually has wheels, which means that it is mobile and you can walk around while the drip is connected to you.

A drip is usually controlled with a pump to keep the fluid flowing into your vein at the right speed. The pump might make a beeping sound from time to time to let the nurses know if something is not right. Don't worry if this happens – the drip stops until the problem is corrected.

Important: Tell the nurses if you feel any discomfort while you are having IV chemotherapy. Occasionally the drug goes into the tissues around the vein instead of into the vein itself. This is called 'extravasation' and can cause damage to the tissues if it isn't stopped quickly. All nurses who give chemotherapy are trained in how to deal with this complication.

IV given through a central venous catheter ('line')

You might have your IV chemotherapy through a central venous catheter ('central line' or 'line'). This is a tube that goes into a bigger vein than a cannula and stays there for a longer amount of time. It can be left in for several months, sometimes even for the whole of your treatment. Lines usually do not cause any pain.

Not everybody needs a line. Sometimes, having a line can make it easier to give you drugs and other fluids and to take blood samples without the discomfort of repeated needle pricks.

Lines are put in during a small operation done under local or general anaesthetic. Once the line is in, you will have a chest X-ray to check that it is in the right position.

There are two types of line:

- **PICC line** (peripherally inserted central catheter), which goes in through a vein in your arm at the level of your elbow. It is held in place by a very secure dressing.
- **Tunnelled central line**, which is usually positioned on your upper chest. Part of it runs in a 'tunnel' under your skin, which lowers the risk of infection. You might also hear this type of line called a Hickman® line, a Groshong® line or apheresis line.

The line is covered to protect it when you go home. You will be given instructions on how to care for it, including on how to manage baths and showers.

Lines can sometimes become infected or can occasionally cause a blood clot to form around them. Contact your hospital immediately if you develop any symptoms of infection, including:

- redness or heat around the line site
- a high temperature (above 38°C)
- arm swelling.

Intrathecal chemotherapy

Intrathecal chemotherapy is given into the fluid that surrounds the central nervous system (CNS; brain and spinal cord). This fluid is called 'cerebrospinal fluid'.

The CNS is surrounded by a blood-brain barrier that protects against infections; however, it also prevents many drugs getting into the CNS through the bloodstream. Only certain drugs can pass through the blood-brain barrier when they are given intravenously. Intrathecal chemotherapy is a way to bypass the blood-brain barrier and give drugs directly into the CNS.

You might have intrathecal chemotherapy if you have:

- Lymphoma in your brain and spinal cord; central nervous system (CNS).
- A type of high-grade lymphoma that can sometimes spread to the CNS (such as Burkitt lymphoma, diffuse large B-cell lymphoma with particular risk features) or lymphoblastic lymphoma. In these cases, you may have intrathecal chemotherapy to prevent the lymphoma from spreading there; this is called 'CNS prophylaxis'.

Intrathecal chemotherapy is usually given by a lumbar puncture. This is an injection into cerebrospinal fluid in the lower part of your back under a local anaesthetic.

Subcutaneous chemotherapy

A small number of chemotherapy drugs are given by injection into the layer of fat that lies just under your skin (subcutaneous chemotherapy). You might have subcutaneous chemotherapy if you are being treated for hairy cell leukaemia (HCL).

Some other types of treatment can be given by subcutaneous injection, for example maintenance rituximab, growth factors and immunoglobulin replacement therapy.

The nurse injects the drug through a tiny needle into the skin on your tummy, upper arm or thigh. The injection is not usually painful but it may sting for a few moments. The time it takes to give the drug depends on what drug you are having.

14.6 What side effects might I have?

Although the aim is to kill lymphoma cells, many types of chemotherapy also temporarily affect healthy cells. This is the reason for many of the side effects of chemotherapy.

Your medical team should advise you on whether they expect you to have side effects during or soon after your treatment. They should also talk to you about any possible late effects you might have. Late effects are health problems that first appear months or years after treatment has finished.

The side effects you have depend on which type of chemotherapy drug you are given and any pre-existing conditions you have. They can also vary a lot between different people having the same treatments.

The side effects listed here are intended as a general guide. You are unlikely to have all of them and you may have only a few. Your medical team should talk through the details and possible side effects of your treatment and give you some written information to take away.

Shorter term common side effects can include:

- Low blood counts – neutropenia (low white blood cells, which can increase your risk of infection), anaemia (low red blood cells, which can make you tired, light-headed, dizzy or breathless) and thrombocytopenia (low platelets, which can increase your risk of infection, bruising or bleeding).
- Fatigue (extreme tiredness), which may come and go in peaks and troughs and worsen after each cycle of treatment.
- Nausea (feeling and being sick) – if your drugs are likely to cause sickness, your medical team may be able to prescribe antiemetics (anti-sickness medication) to help manage it.
- Hair loss or thinning and changes to your nails – many people worry about this; however, not all chemotherapy drugs have this effect and any effects are usually temporary.
- Sore mouth and ulcers – your mouth may become swollen and red a week or two after you start chemotherapy.
- Changes in taste – many people say food tastes bland. Others describe a metallic taste, or find that food tastes more salty or bitter than usual.
- Skin changes including rashes – some drugs make your skin photosensitive (more sensitive to sunlight). The drugs that are more likely to cause this are dacarbazine and methotrexate. Allergic skin reactions and 'papular rash' (small, red rashes) are also common.

- Peripheral neuropathy (effects on some of your nerve endings) and can cause symptoms such as pins and needles, numbness and tingling.
- Changes in bowel habits (such as diarrhoea and constipation).
- Bladder symptoms – cyclophosphamide (particularly in a high dose) and ifosfamide (Mitoxana®) can cause irritation to, and bleeding from the lining of the bladder and the kidneys. You may be given a drug called mesna (Uromitexan®) to prevent bladder and kidney complications.
- Cancer-related cognitive impairment ('chemo brain') – after treatment for lymphoma, some people experience a change in thinking processes, such as difficulty with concentrating or with remembering things.

14.6.1 Other possible side effects

Other possible side effects only occur with particular chemotherapy drugs.

These can include:

- hearing changes, for example temporary loss or tinnitus (ringing in your ears)
- flu-like symptoms
- heart problems
- lung problems.

Your medical team should speak to you before you begin treatment about any side effects you should expect.

14.7 What late effects might I have?

Late effects are health problems that first appear weeks, months or years after treatment has finished. Examples of possible late effects after chemotherapy include heart or lung problems.

Not everyone gets late effects. The late effects you have depend on which chemotherapy drug you have, the strength of the dose and the duration of treatment.

Your doctor should talk to you about possible late effects before you begin treatment.

14.7.1 Effects on fertility

Your fertility (ability to have children) may be affected by treatment. This can range from reduced fertility to loss of fertility, for example through early menopause.

Effects on fertility are more likely with certain chemotherapy drugs and at higher doses, such as those used in stem cell transplants.

You may wish to find out from your medical team about fertility preservation – talk to them before you begin your treatment.

14.7.2 Second cancers

People who have had chemotherapy have a slightly higher risk of developing another form of cancer, including leukaemia, some years later.

Ask your medical team which cancers you are at a higher risk of developing. Make sure you know the symptoms of these cancers – cancer is usually more treatable when it is diagnosed early.

Cancer Research UK has information about different types of cancers. It is important to avoid smoking to reduce the risk of developing other cancers.

14.8 How will I be followed-up after treatment?

After finishing your treatment for lymphoma, you will have regular follow-up appointments at the hospital. These involve conversations and physical tests with a member of your medical team.

One of the tests you are likely to have in the first few months after chemotherapy is the full blood count (FBC). This measures the numbers and sizes of your blood cells and tells doctors how well your bone marrow is working.

The aim of follow-up is to:

- monitor your recovery from treatment
- check for signs of relapse (the lymphoma coming back)
- manage any late effects of treatment.

How often you are followed-up depends on several factors. These include the type of lymphoma you had, how long it's been since you had treatment and whether you were treated as part of a clinical trial.

14.9 Frequently asked questions

Below are some frequently asked questions about chemotherapy for lymphoma. Do not hesitate to ask questions – your medical team are used to going over things and want to help you.

14.9.1 Will I have other treatments together with my chemotherapy?

As well as your chemotherapy drugs you will probably have other drugs to take as part of a chemotherapy regimen, for example:

- steroids, often in the form of prednisolone tablets
- targeted therapies such as antibody therapies (for example rituximab); some of these are in tablet form and others are given by intravenous injection or by subcutaneous injection.

Other treatments may be given to help you with the side effects of chemotherapy.

- G-CSF (granulocyte colony-stimulating factor) is a 'growth factor' given by subcutaneous injection. It helps the bone marrow to make healthy new white blood cells.
- Anti-emetic (anti-sickness) medicines stop you feeling sick. There are several different kinds of anti-emetic drug – tell your nurses or doctors if the drug they give you isn't working so that they can try another one.

14.9.2 Why can't surgery cure my lymphoma?

Surgery can't remove all the cancerous cells in lymphoma. Even for lymphomas that appear to be in one area only, surgery usually leaves some cells behind. For this reason, chemotherapy and/or radiotherapy are the standard treatments.

14.9.3 How can I reduce my risk of infection while I'm having treatment?

You are more prone to infections and may be less able to shake them off while you are on chemotherapy. It is important that you know:

- how to spot the signs of infection
- what to do if you think you might have an infection
- how to lower the risk of infection.

14.9.4 How long do chemotherapy drugs stay in your body?

In most cases, drugs last from a few hours to a few days in the body. It can, however, take longer for them to be completely eliminated.

The length of time a drug stays in your body depends on factors such as the type of drug you are given and how your body processes it. It also depends how well your organs are working, for example your kidneys and liver, as most drugs are excreted through your urine or stools (feaces).

14.9.5 Can I drink alcohol?

Check with your consultant whether it is safe for you to drink alcohol. Alcohol can interact with some drugs and may affect how well they work.

Generally, it should be okay to have the occasional drink between chemotherapy cycles when you feel well enough, but seek medical advice first. Remember, too, that you may feel the effects of alcohol more quickly now than you did before you had treatment.

14.9.6 Can I smoke?

Smoking increases your risk of developing infections, especially in the lungs. If you are currently having treatment for lymphoma, the risk increases further.

Some chemotherapy drugs, including bleomycin, increase the risk of pulmonary fibrosis (scarring in the lungs), which can lead to breathing problems. If you smoke, stopping can help to lower these risks. NHS Choices has information and advice to help you quit smoking.

14.9.7 Is it safe to exercise?

Exercise can have a positive impact on physical and mental health. It may also shorten your recovery time after treatment.

Speak to your doctor about the type and intensity of exercise that's safe for you. They may advise you to avoid certain types of exercise at times. For example, you'll probably be advised to avoid contact sports like rugby if you have thrombocytopenia (low platelets), due to the risk of bruising and bleeding. Swimming may also not be advised for a while because of the increased risk of infection from public pools and changing rooms. It could also dislodge a central line or PICC line.

14.9.8 Am I likely to lose my hair?

Full hair loss is common only with some, not all, types of chemotherapy. Speak to your medical team about what to expect. You may also be interested in suggestions for how to cope with hair loss and in exploring headwear options.

14.9.9 Is it safe to have a massage?

Some people with lymphoma worry that having a massage could spread the lymphoma throughout their body. Little research has been done into massage specifically for people with lymphoma but at the time of writing, there is nothing to say that gentle massage is unsafe. Speak to your medical team for advice if you would like to have a massage.

14.9.10 Could complementary therapies help me?

There is some evidence that acupuncture can help with nausea and vomiting as side effects of chemotherapy. It may also provide some pain relief. As with all complementary therapies, speak to a member of your medical team before you decide whether to have acupuncture – if you have thrombocytopenia or neutropenia, you could be at greater risk of bleeding or infection.

14.9.11 Can I carry on working?

You are likely to need to take some time out of work while you're having treatment for lymphoma and probably for a little while after finishing treatment. You might choose to carry on working through your treatment. Your employer must, by law, make any 'reasonable adjustments' that allow you to continue working during and after treatment (under the Equality Act 2010).

Speak to your HR department or your line-manager and ask how they can support you. You may also be interested in finding out about any sources of financial support available to you if your income is lowered.

Your keyworker (often your Clinical Nurse Specialist; CNS) is often a good person to speak to. He or she may be able to signpost you to further sources of advice and support.

14.9.12 Can I see friends and family?

The support of friends and family can greatly improve your mental wellbeing and might encourage you to take good care of your general health. Be realistic, though, and try not to let people put you under pressure to do more than you want to do socially.

If you have a particular event that you want to attend, such as a family wedding, talk to your medical team. It may be possible to plan your schedule of treatment so that you are likely to feel as well as possible on the day.

14.9.13 Can I have a flu vaccination?

Ask your medical team whether they advise that you have the flu vaccination. The vaccine may not work effectively while you are having chemotherapy and may only be advisable before or after a course of chemotherapy.

It is sensible to have the flu vaccination every year once you have completed your chemotherapy.

14.9.14 Are there any restrictions in what I can eat?

Aim to eat a healthy, balanced diet. Make sure that all fruit and vegetables are well washed, meat and eggs are thoroughly cooked, avoid shellfish, pate, unpasteurised soft cheeses and live yogurts.

If you are having a more intensive chemotherapy regimen, your medical team may give you some additional advice on foods to avoid.

14.9.15 Can I go out in public?

It is fine to go out in public, though you should take care to minimise the risk of infection if you are neutropenic.

14.9.16 Can I have sex?

Generally, sex during treatment is considered to be safe and can enhance your wellbeing. Check with your medical team about any precautions you should take, though, especially if you have thrombocytopenia (low platelets).

During chemotherapy, you should use a condom to avoid passing chemotherapy to your partner and to protect against infection. Note that pregnancy is not recommended during treatment.

Oral contraceptive tablets ('the pill') may be less effective while you are on treatment, so discuss this with your doctor or nurse – you may need to use a different form of contraception for a while.

14.9.17 When can I get pregnant after my treatment?

Your fertility may be reduced by the chemotherapy. Your medical team should discuss this possibility with you before you start treatment.

Whether your fertility is likely to be reduced by your treatment or not, it is not a good idea to start a pregnancy while you are on chemotherapy or soon afterwards. Women are strongly advised to wait for two years after their treatment for lymphoma has finished before trying to start a family. Men with lymphoma are usually advised that they should avoid making their partner pregnant during their chemotherapy and for at least six months afterwards.

Talk to your hospital team for fertility advice specific to your individual circumstances.

14.9.18 Can I breastfeed while I am having treatment?

Chemotherapy drugs may be present in your breast milk so you should avoid breastfeeding your baby during treatment. Ask your doctor for further information.

14.9.19 Can I go on holiday when I am having chemotherapy?

Most doctors would not recommend travelling abroad outside of the UK during chemotherapy and for three months afterwards.

Short breaks in the UK are usually fine so long as you feel well enough and have access to a hospital if needed.

15 Chemotherapy regimens for lymphoma

Chemotherapy regimens (combinations of drugs) for lymphoma. We have separate information about chemotherapy, including how it works, how it is given and its possible side effects.

15.1 What is a chemotherapy regimen?

A regimen is a plan of treatment that involves drugs such as chemotherapy. A regimen specifies:

- the name of the drug or drugs you will have
- the dose of each drug
- how often you take them
- how long you take each drug for.

Most regimens are given as a block of chemotherapy followed by a rest period to allow your body to recover. This is known as a 'cycle'. Your medical team will talk to you about how many treatment cycles you need.

Many chemotherapy regimens include a combination of drugs. Each drug works in a slightly different way to kill the lymphoma cells. Together, the drugs can kill more of the lymphoma.

Some chemotherapy drugs may be given on their own (for example pixantrone and bendamustine), especially if the aim of treatment is to control symptoms of lymphoma.

Chemotherapy drugs are sometimes given with a different type of drug, such as an antibody therapy like rituximab, a targeted drug like ibrutinib, or a steroid such as prednisolone.

15.2 Common chemotherapy regimens for lymphoma

On this page we list the most common chemotherapy regimens for lymphoma.

The names of chemotherapy regimens are usually acronyms made up of the first letters of each of the drugs they contain. Sometimes, to make them easier to say, a regimen uses a drug's 'trade' or brand name (the name the pharmaceutical company gives the drug). Trade names start with a capital letter and are sometimes followed by a registered trademark (®).

Some chemotherapy regimens aren't referred to by acronyms. These include bendamustine and chlorambucil, which may be used in combination with rituximab to treat certain types of lymphoma.

Antibody therapies, such as rituximab, or targeted drugs, such as ibrutinib, are sometimes given on their own or with chemotherapy for some types of lymphoma. When rituximab is added to a chemotherapy regimen, an 'R' is added to the name – for example R-CHOP, R-ICE, R-CVP and R-bendamustine. Rituximab is usually used only for B-cell non-Hodgkin lymphomas.

15.2.1 Acronyms for chemotherapy regimens sometimes used to treat lymphoma

ABVD – **d**oxorubicin
(**A**driamycin®), **b**leomycin, **v**inblastine and **d**acarbazine

BEACOPP – **b**leomycin, **e**toposide, doxorubicin
(**A**driamycin®), **c**yclophosphamide, vincristine
(**O**ncovin®), **p**rocarbazine and **p**rednisolone; a higher-dose regimen is sometimes called BEACOPPesc (escalated dose)

BEAM – carmustine (**B**iCNU®), **e**toposide, cytarabine
(**A**ra-C) and **m**elphalan

CHEOP – **c**yclophosmamide, doxorubicin
(or **h**ydroxydaunorubicin), **e**toposide, vincristine
(**O**ncovin®) and **p**rednisolone

ChlVPP – **chl**orambucil, **v**inblastine, **p**rocarbazine
and **p**rednisolone

CHOP – **c**yclophosphamide, doxorubicin
(or **h**ydroxydaunorubicin), vincristine (**O**ncovin®)
and **p**rednisolone

CHVPi – **c**yclophosphamide, doxorubicin
(or **h**ydroxydaunorubicin), etoposide
(**V**epesid®), **p**rednisolone and **i**nterferon-alpha

CODOX-M – **c**yclophosphamide, vincristine (**O**ncovin®), **d**oxorubicin and **m**ethotrexate

CVP – **c**yclophosphamide, **v**incristine and **p**rednisolone

DA-EPOCH – **d**ose-**a**djusted **e**toposide, **p**rednisolone, vincristine (**O**ncovin®), **c**yclophosphamide and doxorubicin (or **h**ydroxydaunorubicin)

DHAP – **d**examethasone, **h**igh-dose cytarabine (**A**ra-C) and cisplatin (**P**latinol®)

ESHAP – **e**toposide, methylprednisolone (**S**olu-Medrone®), **h**igh-dose cytarabine (**A**ra-C) and cisplatin (**P**latinol®)

FC – **f**ludarabine and **c**yclophosphamide

GCVP – **g**emcitabine, **c**yclophosphamide, **v**incristine and **p**rednisolone

GDP – **g**emcitabine, **d**examethasone and cisplatin (**P**latinol®)

GEMOX – **gem**citabine and **ox**aliplatin

GEM-P – **gem**citabine, cisplatin and methyl**p**rednisolone

Hyper-CVAD – **c**yclophosphamide, **v**incristine, doxorubicin (**A**driamycin®) and **d**examethasone; 'hyper' is short for 'hyperfractionated', which means that you have the same drug more than once in a day

ICE – **i**fosfamide, **c**arboplatin and **e**toposide

IGEV – **i**fosfamide, **g**emcitabine and **v**inorelbine

IVAC – **i**fosfamide, etoposide (**V**P-16) and cytarabine (**A**ra-C)

Maxi-CHOP – **maxi**mum dose **c**yclophosphamide, doxorubicin (or **h**ydroxydaunorubicin), vincristine (**O**ncovin®) and **p**rednisolone

MCP – **m**itoxantrone, **c**hlorambucil and **p**rednisolone
P-
MitCEBO – **p**rednisolone, **mit**oxantrone, **c**yclophosphamide, **e**toposide, **b**leomycin and vincristine (**O**ncovin®)

15.3 Which chemotherapy regimen might I have?

The exact regimen you have depends on a number of factors including:

- the type of lymphoma you have
- how quickly the lymphoma is growing – whether it's fast-growing (high-grade) or slow-growing (low-grade)
- where in your body the lymphoma is
- the symptoms or problems that your lymphoma is causing
- whether you have previously had other treatments for lymphoma
- if you have any other health conditions or you are taking any other medicines
- your age, general health and fitness.

Your medical team will talk to you about the best treatment for you based on your individual circumstances.

15.4 Side effects of chemotherapy regimens

Treatment affects each person differently. Your doctor, clinical nurse specialist or chemotherapy nurse should speak to you about any side effects and late effects you might expect from your chemotherapy regimen.

Macmillan Cancer Support has an online tool where you can search for a chemotherapy regimen and find out more about it, including its possible side effects.

16 CNS prophylaxis

Treatment given to prevent lymphoma spreading to your central nervous system (CNS) is called 'CNS prophylaxis'. Most people with lymphoma do not need this type of treatment. Your doctor might recommend this preventative treatment if you have certain types of lymphoma or risk factors that could put you at higher risk of your lymphoma spreading to your CNS (brain, spinal cord and eyes).

16.1 What is CNS prophylaxis?

'Prophylaxis' is a treatment that is designed to prevent something. Central nervous system (CNS) prophylaxis is treatment that aims to stop lymphoma spreading to the brain and spinal cord.

Some types of lymphoma can spread to the CNS from somewhere else.

Many chemotherapy regimens (combinations of drugs; for example CHOP) do not reach the CNS. The lymphoma might be treated successfully elsewhere, but tiny numbers of cells could be present in your CNS and could continue to grow. This can cause the lymphoma to relapse (come back) in your CNS.

Lymphoma that is in the CNS but started somewhere else is known as 'secondary CNS lymphoma'. It can be difficult to treat secondary CNS lymphoma and it can cause long-term neurological (brain and nerve) problems, so doctors sometimes suggest giving treatment to prevent it developing.

Most people with lymphoma have a low risk of secondary CNS lymphoma and do not need CNS prophylaxis. Your medical team will only suggest CNS prophylaxis if you have risk factors that make your lymphoma more likely to spread to the CNS.

You do not have CNS prophylaxis if there is evidence that your lymphoma is already in your CNS.

What is the central nervous system?

The central nervous system (CNS) is the part of your body that controls all your body's functions. It includes the brain, the spinal cord and the eyes.

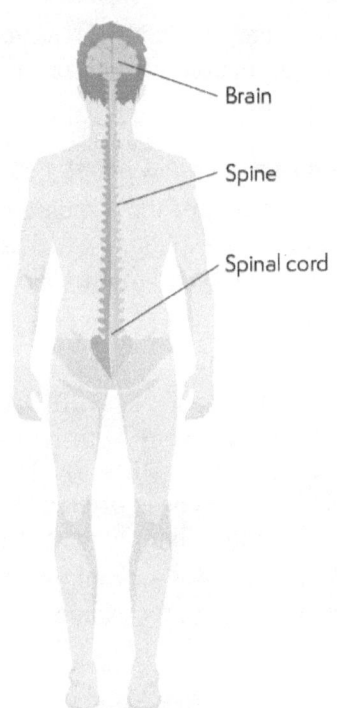

Figure: The brain and spinal cord

Your CNS is protected from the rest of your body.

- A special fluid called 'cerebrospinal fluid' (CSF) surrounds the brain and spinal cord to cushion them.
- The blood-brain barrier surrounds your brain. It is a barrier of cells and blood vessels that only lets certain substances reach the brain to protect it from harmful chemicals and infections.

It is important that your CNS is protected from harm. However, this protection can make it difficult to treat lymphoma in this area.

16.2 Who might need CNS prophylaxis?

CNS prophylaxis is part of the standard treatment for very fast-growing types of lymphoma, which are the most likely types of lymphoma to spread to the CNS. For example:

- Burkitt lymphoma
- lymphoblastic lymphoma.

Diffuse large B-cell lymphoma (DLBCL) can spread to the CNS. However, not everyone with DLBCL has the same risk. Most people with DLBCL do not need CNS prophylaxis. This treatment is offered only to people who have a higher risk of their lymphoma spreading to the CNS.

You are likely to have CNS prophylaxis if DLBCL is in certain areas of your body, for example, in a:

- testicle
- breast
- adrenal gland (glands that produce hormones to help your body function correctly)
- kidney.

You might also be at higher risk of lymphoma spreading to your CNS if the lymphoma is growing close to it, for example at the base of your skull or around your spine.

You might also have CNS prophylaxis if you have several of the following factors that can increase your risk of lymphoma affecting your CNS. The more of these risk factors you have, the greater the risk of lymphoma spreading to your CNS. Your doctor is likely to recommend CNS prophylaxis if you have four or five of these risk factors, and will consider whether you need CNS prophylaxis if you have two or three risk factors:

- you have high levels of a chemical called 'lactate dehydrogenase (LDH)' in your blood
- you are over 60 years old
- you are particularly unwell when first diagnosed with lymphoma
- your lymphoma is in two or more extranodal sites (two or more places outside of the lymph nodes)
- you have stage 3 or 4 DLBCL.

Many doctors use the same markers of higher risk when treating people with other types of high-grade non-Hodgkin lymphoma, including primary mediastinal large B-cell lymphoma, some types of T-cell lymphoma and transformation of low-grade lymphoma into a faster-growing type of lymphoma.

People with mantle cell lymphoma do not usually need CNS prophylaxis. Your doctor might suggest CNS prophylaxis if they think you could be at higher risk of secondary CNS lymphoma.

It is very uncommon for secondary CNS lymphoma to develop in people with low-grade non-Hodgkin lymphoma or Hodgkin lymphoma. People with these types of lymphoma very rarely need CNS prophylaxis.

Speak to your medical team if you are concerned about your risk of developing secondary CNS lymphoma and whether CNS prophylaxis is suitable for you. Your medical team are best placed to advise you on whether you need CNS prophylaxis. They can also explain the risks and benefits of this type of treatment.

16.3 How is CNS prophylaxis given?

The brain is protected from harmful chemicals and infections by the blood–brain barrier: a barrier of cells and blood vessels that only lets certain substances through. Depending on whether a drug can cross the blood–brain barrier, CNS prophylaxis can be given in two ways:

- intrathecal chemotherapy for drugs that can't cross the blood–brain barrier
- intravenous chemotherapy for drugs that can cross the blood–brain barrier.

You might be given CNS prophylaxis by either or both methods. It is difficult for doctors to find out which type of CNS prophylaxis works best as secondary CNS lymphoma is uncommon.

16.3.1 Intrathecal chemotherapy

Intrathecal chemotherapy is where chemotherapy is given directly into the CSF. This method avoids the blood–brain barrier so chemotherapy can reach your CNS. It also means the additional chemotherapy only affects your CNS and not the rest of your body.

The chemotherapy is usually injected during a lumbar puncture.

Only certain drugs can be safely given intrathecally (into the CSF). The most common drug given intrathecally for CNS prophylaxis is methotrexate. For CNS prophylaxis, intrathecal methotrexate is usually given once during each cycle of standard chemotherapy.

You are likely to have fewer side effects if drugs are given intrathecally than if they are given intravenously. Side effects might include:

- nausea and vomiting
- headache (this is common after a lumbar puncture)
- fever.

Rarely, more serious side effects can occur if CSF leaks from the injection site or if there is any damage to your CNS during or following the procedure.

Cancer Research UK have more information on methotrexate, including information on side effects.

Intravenous chemotherapy

Certain drugs can cross the blood-brain barrier when given intravenously (into a vein). The most common drug given intravenously as CNS prophylaxis is high-dose methotrexate.

Intravenous methotrexate for CNS prophylaxis is given as an infusion (drip). It typically takes 3 to 4 hours for the drug to be given. You have to stay in hospital for a few days as you need to have lots of fluids before and after the drug is given. This reduces the risk of side effects. Common side effects include:

- Problems due to too much fluid circulating in your body. This can cause breathlessness and swelling.
- Problems with kidney function. This is usually temporary and recovers but occasionally, serious problems can develop, which can be ongoing.
- Problems with liver function. This is usually temporary and recovers but very rarely, serious problems can develop.

Other intravenous drugs that can be used as CNS prophylaxis include cytarabine and ifosphamide. These drugs are both included in the standard treatment for Burkitt lymphoma. The intensive regimens used for Burkitt lymphoma are sometimes used for people with DLBCLwhen doctors think it might not respond well to the usual treatment, R-CHOP. Cytarabine is used as part of the standard treatment for people with mantle cell lymphoma who are fit enough for intensive treatment.

Your medical team should explain to you which side effects you can expect depending on the drugs you are having and your individual circumstances.

17 Radiotherapy

radiotherapy treatment for lymphoma.

17.1 Quick overview

Radiotherapy is a treatment that uses radiation to destroy cancer cells.

17.1.1 What is the aim of radiotherapy?

You might have radiotherapy with the aim of curing your lymphoma (curative radiotherapy) or to control your symptoms (palliative radiotherapy). Not everyone who has lymphoma has radiotherapy.

17.1.2 How often will I have treatment and how long does it take?

A course of radiotherapy usually involves an initial 'planning session'. Treatment then usually starts on a different day. Your doctor decides how many treatments ('fractions') of radiotherapy you should have; this can vary from a single treatment, to treatment 5 days a week over 3-4 weeks. You usually have it once a day, Monday to Friday, with a rest at the weekend.

17.1.3 Is radiotherapy painful?

You cannot feel radiotherapy; it is painless.

17.1.4 What are the side effects of radiotherapy?

It is quite common to feel tired after radiotherapy. Other side effects depend on the area of your body that is treated with radiotherapy and the type of radiotherapy you have.

17.2 What is radiotherapy?

Radiotherapy uses high energy X-rays and other types of radiation. The treatment has been used successfully to treat lymphoma for over 50 years.

17.2.1 How does radiotherapy work?

Lymphoma is a type of cancer. It develops when lymphocytes (specialised white blood cells) grow out of control and build up in the lymph nodes and other organs. This can happen when lymphocytes divide more often than normal. It can also happen when they do not die when they should.

Radiotherapy causes damage to lymphoma cells in the treated area, which means that they die off with time. Although surrounding healthy cells can also be affected by radiotherapy, they can repair themselves and recover. Lymphoma cells are much more sensitive to radiotherapy than most other types of cancer cell. The dose of radiation needed to treat lymphoma is therefore relatively low, so side effects are often mild.

Radiotherapy is a local treatment, which means it only affects the part or parts of the body being treated. Radiotherapy is painless and does not make you radioactive.

17.3 Radiotherapy for lymphoma

You might have radiotherapy with the aim of curing your lymphoma or to control your symptoms.

17.3.1 Radiotherapy to cure lymphoma (curative radiotherapy)

Radiotherapy is often used with the aim of curing the lymphoma by destroying all of it.

Depending on which type and stage of lymphoma you have, your treatment might involve radiotherapy alone, or a combination of chemotherapy and radiotherapy.

- Some types of lymphoma that are low grade or 'indolent' (slow-growing) can be cured with radiotherapy alone if they are at an early stage.
- High-grade lymphomas that are early stage are often treated with chemotherapy followed by radiotherapy.
- High-grade lymphomas that are at a more advanced stage are usually treated with chemotherapy. You may also have some radiotherapy after finishing your chemotherapy.

17.3.2 Radiotherapy to control symptoms of lymphoma (palliative radiotherapy)

Sometimes, radiotherapy is used to control symptoms such as pain and discomfort. This is known as 'palliative radiotherapy'. It helps by reducing the size of the lymphoma.

17.3.3 When will I have radiotherapy?

Radiotherapy might be your only treatment, or you might have it after chemotherapy.

When both chemotherapy and radiotherapy are used, the aim is that:

- Chemotherapy treats the main area of the lymphoma. It also destroys small clusters of lymphoma cells that are some way away from the main site (area) of the disease.
- Radiotherapy then targets the main site of the lymphoma. With curative radiotherapy, this aims to increase the likelihood that the lymphoma is completely destroyed.

It is unusual for a lymphoma to relapse (come back) in a part of the body that has already been treated with curative radiotherapy.

17.3.4 Which types of lymphoma does radiotherapy treat?

Radiotherapy for Hodgkin lymphoma

You might be treated with radiotherapy if you have:

- Classical Hodgkin lymphoma that is at an early stage, after a course of chemotherapy.

- Advanced Hodgkin lymphoma, sometimes if there are very enlarged (bulky) lymph nodes or areas that seem not to have completely responded to chemotherapy.
- Nodular lymphocyte-predominant Hodgkin lymphoma (NLPHL) that is at an early stage. In these cases, radiotherapy alone is often recommended.

Radiotherapy for non-Hodgkin lymphoma

Radiotherapy is used to treat many types of non-Hodgkin lymphoma. You might be treated with radiotherapy if you have a:

- Low-grade or 'indolent' (slow-growing) non-Hodgkin lymphoma, such as follicular lymphoma or marginal zone lymphoma. In these cases, it can be used if the lymphoma is localised to just one area with the aim of cure. If the lymphoma is more widespread, palliative radiotherapy might be used to control symptoms.
- High-grade or 'aggressive' (fast-growing) types, such as diffuse large B-cell lymphoma (DLBCL). If the lymphoma is at an early stage, treatment often involves a course of chemotherapy followed by radiotherapy. If the lymphoma is more advanced, chemotherapy is usually given. Nonetheless, radiotherapy can be used after chemotherapy to treat areas of lymphoma that were large before chemotherapy. It may also be given after chemotherapy to areas that may not have responded completely to chemotherapy.

17.4 What types of radiotherapy are there?

The type of radiotherapy and length of treatment depends on where the lymphoma is and the aim of the radiotherapy.

Most radiotherapy is given by high energy X-rays (photons). These are produced by a linear accelerator (Linac) machine and can be given in different ways, including:

- single beams
- multiple beams
- intensity modulated radiotherapy (IMRT), which shapes the dose delivered using lots of beams.

Your clinical oncologist (a doctor who specialises in the treatment of cancer) chooses the most appropriate method for you.

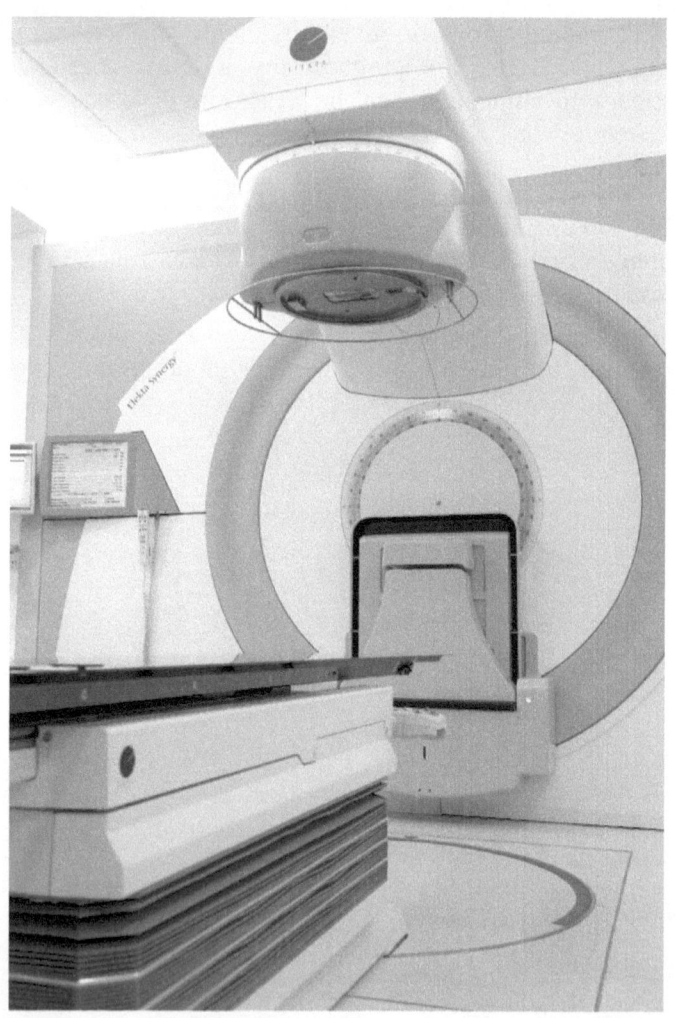

Figure: Radiotherapy machine. Image courtesy of Leeds Teaching Hospitals NHS Trust

Sometimes, if the lymphoma is on the skin or near the surface, electron beam therapy may be recommended. Electrons are tiny particles of radiation that are unable to travel very far in the body. This keeps them to within a short distance under the skin, which means that they cannot affect tissues that are deeper than this.

Electrons are produced by a linear accelerator machine that has an 'applicator' connected to the head of the machine. The applicator directs electrons to the area of your body that is to be treated. When the machine is set up, the applicator is brought very close to you and may even touch you. You won't feel anything during the treatment, though.

Two types of radiotherapy are occasionally used in particular circumstances: total body irradiation (TBI) and total skin electron therapy (TSET).

17.4.1 Total body irradiation (TBI)

Total body irradiation (TBI) is a type of high energy X-ray radiotherapy that is delivered to the whole body.

If you need an allogeneic (donor) stem cell transplant, you might have TBI as part of your conditioning treatment before the procedure. This helps to destroy your own bone marrow (a part of larger bones, where blood cells are made). In doing so, space is made for the healthy new stem cells, which stops you rejecting the transplant.

TBI can be given as a single dose or twice a day over several days. Your radiotherapy team should talk you through your treatment plan.

17.4.2 Total skin electron radiotherapy (TSET)

Total skin electron radiotherapy (TSET) is a specialised technique for skin lymphoma. Electrons are used to treat the whole skin surface. There are different ways of doing this. Your doctor should explain which technique is best for you.

17.5 Where will I have radiotherapy?

You need to go to hospital for your treatment to be planned and each time you are given radiotherapy.

You may have to travel for radiotherapy if your local hospital does not have a radiotherapy department. Not all hospitals have a radiotherapy department because the equipment is very expensive and requires a dedicated treatment room. Staff members giving radiotherapy are also highly specialised.

Radiotherapy for lymphoma is usually given Monday to Friday. The length of treatment can vary from a single day to 4 weeks. Don't worry if your schedule differs from this – your treatment plan is designed specifically for you and your medical team will talk you through it beforehand.

17.6 How much radiotherapy will I need?

The total dose of radiotherapy, measured in Gray (Gy), is split into separate treatments or 'fractions'. Highly trained specialists calculate the right dose of radiation for you.

Palliative radiotherapy can be very effective when given in just one fraction; however, it might be given over a longer course.

Curative radiotherapy is usually given over a few weeks and treatment sessions are spread out to give healthy cells a chance to repair between treatments. Giving treatment in fractions also increases the likelihood of the treatment reaching the lymphoma cells at a time when they are most sensitive to radiotherapy.

Modern techniques and knowledge mean that it is possible to use a much lower total dose of radiotherapy and to target lymphoma cells more accurately than in the past. This reduces the side effects caused by radiation to healthy cells. At the same time, it allows successful treatment of the lymphoma.

17.7 How is radiotherapy planned?

Radiotherapy needs careful planning. This is to make it is as effective as possible and to minimise side effects.

When you and your medical team have decided on radiotherapy, you are under the care of a clinical oncologist.

During planning, the radiotherapy team make sure that the right amount of radiotherapy is delivered to precisely the right place. They look at:

- exactly where the lymphoma is – this area will receive the most of your total dose of radiotherapy
- the area around the lymphoma – this area may receive a smaller amount of radiotherapy if there is a risk that some lymphoma cells have spread there
- organs at risk – critical structures in the body (such as the brain, heart, and salivary glands). Your treatment is planned to protect these organs from radiation in order to prevent damage to them.

You won't receive radiotherapy to the rest of your body unless you are having total body irradiation (TBI).

17.7.1 How your radiotherapy is planned

You may first have a radiotherapy mask made to help keep you in the same position for each treatment.

For most treatments, radiotherapy is planned with a computed tomography (CT) simulator scan (also known as a 'CT planning scan'). This transfers images to a radiotherapy planning system to help plan your radiotherapy.

For some treatments (usually electron treatments), after you have been positioned ready for treatment, your doctor might use a felt-tipped-like pen to mark the area to be treated.

When you have the CT simulator scan, marks are often made on your skin (unless you are being treated for lymphoma in the head and neck area). Some of these are made using ink, with a felt-tipped-like pen. You may also need a few permanent marks ('tattoos') – usually two or three tiny dots of ink just under the surface of your skin. When you have your treatment, the marks are lined up with the X-ray beams on the treatment machine to make sure the radiotherapy goes to exactly the right place. You might also be given an injection of a 'contrast agent' (dye) through a drip into one of your veins, which helps your doctor to plan your treatment.

The CT simulator scan is used to make a detailed 3D map. The map shows where the lymphoma is and the exact positions of nearby tissues and organs. This information is given to your clinical oncologist and to the radiotherapy physics team. Using computer software, they work out how best to direct the X-ray beams to treat the lymphoma while keeping radiation to nearby parts of the body low. They work within limits of radiation that are known to be safe.

A clinical oncologist approves the radiotherapy treatment plan.

In some hospitals, you may have a practice or 'dummy run' to allow the radiotherapy team to check the treatment before you are given it.

When you have your treatment, the marks are lined up with the X-ray beams on the treatment machine. This is to ensure that the radiotherapy goes to exactly the right place.

17.7.2 Treatment shell or mask

If you have radiotherapy treatment for lymphoma in the head and neck area, you will probably have a thin plastic shell or mask made. The mask helps to get you into the same position each time you have treatment and also helps to keep you still during each treatment.

The shell is usually made from a sheet of thermoplastic. The thermoplastic is softened in warm water for a couple of minutes to make it mouldable. The sheet is then gently laid over your face. You need to stay still while it cools and sets into the shape of your face – this doesn't take long and most people say it doesn't feel unpleasant.

After your shell is made, the radiographers make marks on it to line the radiotherapy beams up with. This ensures that the radiotherapy goes to exactly the right place.

The thought of wearing a shell might seem daunting but most people find it OK, even if they feel nervous beforehand. Holes in the shell over your mouth allow you to breathe easily and often extra holes can be cut out over your eyes and nose. Staff will try to make you feel as comfortable as possible. If you are worried about wearing a mask, let your medical team know. They are very used to this and can give you suggestions to help you feel more relaxed.

17.8 What happens during a radiotherapy session?

You are treated by a radiographer using a linear accelerator machine. This produces high-energy X-ray beams, which deliver an accurate dose of radiation inside the body.

The total time for each treatment session is typically about 10–20 minutes. Most of this time is spent getting you into the correct position to receive the radiotherapy.

17.8.1 Setting up

- You will be in a linear accelerator room, usually lying down on a couch. Staff will take time to get your positioning exactly right. They will check that you are comfortable and that you know what to expect.

- The lights will be dimmed. You will probably notice a beam of light coming from the head of the machine. There will also be some coloured laser beams that come from different points around the room. Laser beams are not harmful. They guide the radiographer to get you and the machine into the correct position.

17.8.2 Having your radiotherapy

The radiographers turn on the lights fully and then leave the room. They then turn on the machine.

- From outside the room, the radiographers watch you on closed-circuit television (CCTV). They can see and hear you the whole time, and you will be able to hear them, too.

- The radiation is given for only a few minutes. The machine makes a whirring noise but you don't feel anything.

Sometimes the radiographers take X-ray or CT images during the treatment session. These are to ensure you are in the correct position – they are not to check that the treatment is working.

- You should feel fine immediately after the treatment and the radiographers will come back into the room to help you up.

17.9 What side effects might I have?

Your medical team should advise you on whether they expect you to have side effects during or soon after your treatment. They should also talk to you about any possible late effects you might have. Late effects are health problems that first appear weeks, months or years after treatment has finished.

The side effects you experience depend on which area of your body is treated and the type of radiotherapy you have. Generally, other than tiredness, radiotherapy only causes side effects in the area being treated.

The side effects listed here are intended as a general guide. Please note, however, that the side effects you experience will depend upon which part of your body is being treated and the dose of radiotherapy you have.

Shorter term side effects can include:
- fatigue
- sore skin
- sore mouth
- nausea
- diarrhoea

- hair loss.

17.9.1 Fatigue

Most people feel tired after radiotherapy. You may even experience fatigue – an extreme tiredness that doesn't go away after rest or sleep. Fatigue can be difficult to cope with, both physically and emotionally. There are things you can do to help. It may also be helpful to arrange for a friend or relative to provide you with transport to and from the hospital each time you have treatment.

17.9.2 Sore skin

Some people experience temporary changes to the skin around the treatment area after radiotherapy, which can include:

- soreness that feels a bit like sunburn
- darkening of the skin
- reddening of the skin.

Whether you have sore skin depends on the natural sensitivity of your skin and the area of your body treated. Generally, any changes to your skin improve within a few weeks after finishing treatment.

If your skin becomes very sore during treatment, or if you have a reaction that leads to blistering, your medical team might advise that you have a short break from treatment to allow your skin to recover.

There are lots of things you can do to help with sore skin. You can also ask your medical team about how best to care for your skin during and after radiotherapy treatment.

17.9.3 Sore mouth and throat/discomfort swallowing (mucositis)

Mucositis happens when the mucous membrane (soft tissue that lines the inside of your mouth and throat) becomes inflamed (swollen, red and painful). This can cause pain when swallowing and mouth ulcers (sores). Sore mouth and throat is more common after radiotherapy to the head and neck, particularly at high doses. It typically occurs a couple of weeks after you begin treatment. The risk of sore mouth and throat increases if you are have radiotherapy after chemotherapy.

Sore mouth and throat usually recovers once you finish your treatment, but it can take several weeks.

Ask your medical team how they can help if you have a sore mouth. There are also some simple measures you can take to help relieve pain.

17.9.4 Nausea (feeling sick)

You may feel sick during or for a little while after having radiotherapy and you might actually be sick. Nausea is more likely if the area of your body being treated is around your stomach.

Let your medical team know if you experience nausea – they may be able to prescribe anti-emetics (medication to stop you from feeling sick). There are some simple things you can try to help reduce nausea, too.

17.9.5 Diarrhoea

If you have radiotherapy to the abdominal (stomach) or pelvic area, you might experience diarrhoea. This usually begins several days after starting treatment with radiotherapy and can last for a few weeks.

If you have diarrhoea, tell a member of your medical team so that they can help you to manage it. They may prescribe medication or suggest some steps you can take that may help.

17.9.6 Hair loss

As radiotherapy is given only to a precise area of the body, you will only lose hair from this area.

In general, hair loss happens gradually towards the end of radiotherapy treatment, although it varies from one person to another.

It usually takes around 6–12 months for hair to grow back after treatment has finished. For a small number of people, hair loss in the area treated with radiotherapy is permanent.

17.10 What late effects might I have?

Late effects are health problems that first appear weeks, months or years after treatment has finished.

Not everyone gets late effects. The late effects you have depend on which area of the body was treated with radiotherapy. Your doctor should talk to you about possible late effects before you begin treatment.

17.10.1 Dental problems

Radiotherapy to the head and neck can increase your risk of tooth decay later. Have regular check-ups with your dentist and follow their advice to keep your teeth healthy.

17.10.2 Eye problems

If you've had radiotherapy to an area that includes your eyes, you might have dry eyes. This can be a short-term or a permanent problem. Ask your doctor if there are any treatments that could help. You are also at increased risk of developing cataracts (cloudy patches in the lens of your eye that reduce your vision) in the future. Have regular check-ups with your optician as your prescription may change slightly during treatment and for a short while afterwards.

17.10.3 Heart problems

Radiotherapy can increase the risk of heart problems years later if your heart is in or near the treated area. To minimise this risk, it is sensible to avoid smoking and keep to a healthy lifestyle.

17.10.4 Mouth dryness

This can occur if your salivary glands are treated and depending upon the radiotherapy dose can be a long term effect.

17.10.5 Reduced fertility

There is a risk of infertility if the testes or ovaries are close to the area treated with radiotherapy. This can happen when treatment is given near to the scrotum for men, and near to the pelvis for both men and women. Your doctor will advise if this is the case.

It is important to note that even if there is a risk of an effect on your fertility, radiotherapy does not guarantee infertility; you should use a reliable method of contraception during and for some time after radiotherapy – your medical team will advise you for how long.

If you are of (or younger than) reproductive age, talk to your medical team about preserving your fertility before you begin treatment.

17.10.6 Risk of developing a cancer related to radiotherapy

There is a small risk that radiotherapy can cause a cancer to develop in or near the treated area years later; however, this is rare. Ask your medical team which cancers you are at a higher risk of developing. Make sure you know the symptoms of these cancers – cancer is usually more treatable when it is diagnosed early. Cancer Research UK has information about different types of cancers. It is important to avoid smoking to reduce the risk of developing other cancers.

17.10.7 Lung problems

Radiotherapy to the chest can cause inflammation or scarring to part of your lungs, which can lead to a cough or shortness of breath. Your radiotherapy will be planned to keep this risk as low as possible. It's particularly important not to smoke if you have had radiotherapy to the lungs.

17.10.8 Thyroid problems

Radiotherapy to the neck or upper chest can affect your thyroid gland, which may then make less of the hormone thyroxine. This is called 'hypothyroidism' and can slow your metabolism (the speed at which your body uses energy). Hypothyroidism can make you feel cold and tired, and make you gain weight easily.

The risk of developing hypothyroidism is higher in the first five years after treatment but remains increased after this time. Hypothyroidism is usually picked up early by regular thyroid function blood tests. If you have hypothyroidism, your doctor can prescribe thyroxine tablets to treat it.

You should have regular thyroid function tests. Tell any doctors treating you that you have had treatment for lymphoma so that they are aware of your increased risk of thyroid problems.

17.11 How will I be followed-up after treatment?

After finishing your treatment for lymphoma, you will have regular follow-up appointments at the hospital. These involve conversations and physical tests with a member of your medical team.

The aim of follow-up is to:

- monitor your recovery from treatment
- check for signs of relapse (the lymphoma coming back)
- manage any late effects of treatment.

How often you are followed-up depends on several factors. These include the type of lymphoma you had, how long it's been since you had treatment and whether you were treated as part of a clinical trial.

17.12 Frequently asked questions

Below are some frequently asked questions about radiotherapy. You may find it reassuring to know that radiotherapy is closely supervised by highly skilled radiographers who should explain everything as you go through the process; however, do not hesitate to ask questions – your medical team are used to going over things and want to help you.

17.12.1 Will radiotherapy make me radioactive?

Radiotherapy will not make you radioactive. Those around you, including children, are not at any risk from being near to you after you have had treatment.

17.12.2 Can I take someone into the room with me when I have radiotherapy?

It can be helpful to take someone with you to the hospital for emotional support. However, friends or family members are asked to wait outside the treatment room.

17.12.3 Can I call for attention during treatment if I need to?

Your radiography team can see and hear you the whole time during treatment; you will be able to hear them, too. You can call for attention simply by asking for it or by raising a hand.

17.12.4 Is it safe to have radiotherapy if I have a pacemaker (cardiac rhythm device)?

Generally, people who have a pacemaker can have radiotherapy. However, the radiation can affect how the pacemaker works. Your medical team will carefully monitor you during your treatment to ensure that it works as it should.

17.12.5 Is it safe to have radiotherapy while I am pregnant?

Doctors may wait until after you have given birth before giving you radiotherapy. If you require treatment urgently, they might advise you to go ahead with treatment while taking suitable precautions.

17.12.6 Can I breastfeed if I am having radiotherapy?

Speak to your doctor if you are breastfeeding or plan to breastfeed and radiotherapy has been recommended for you. The safety of breastfeeding depends on which areas of your body receive treatment and the type of radiotherapy you have.

Note: if you are also having drug treatment (such as chemotherapy), you may be advised not to breastfeed during and for a while after treatment.

We have more information about treatment for lymphoma during pregnancy.

18 Antibody therapy for lymphoma (including rituximab)

What antibody therapy is and how it is used to treat lymphoma.

18.1 What are antibodies?

Antibodies are made by the body's immune system and are an important part of its defence against infection. All cells have different proteins on their surface, which are known as antigens. Antibodies bind (stick) to antigens on cells that don't belong in your body, for example on viruses or bacteria cells. If your immune system detects cells that don't belong in your body, it can produce lots of different antibodies. A particular antibody fits only with a particular antigen, like two parts of a jigsaw. When they are bound to an antigen, antibodies attract other cells of the immune system that help to destroy the cells that don't belong in your body.

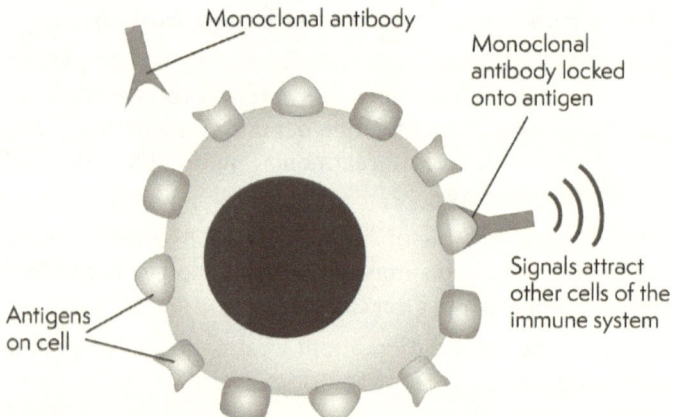

Figure: Monoclonal antibodies locking on to the antigens of a cell

You may hear the term 'monoclonal antibodies'. 'Monoclonal' means that the antibodies are exactly the same, so they stick to exactly the same antigen.

18.2 What is antibody therapy?

Antibody therapy involves giving antibodies that have been specially made in a laboratory to target an antigen on a cancer cell. It is sometimes known as 'immunotherapy' because it helps the body's immune system to recognise and respond to the cancer.

Antibody therapy is a type of targeted therapy. Targeted therapy aims to affect lymphoma cells more precisely than chemotherapy and radiotherapy, reducing the effects on normal cells. Damage to normal cells, such as cells in the bone marrow (the spongy tissue in the centre of some of the large bones of the body where blood cells are made), hair follicles and gut, causes many of the side effects of chemotherapy and radiotherapy.

18.3 How does antibody therapy work?

Antibody therapy can work in different ways.

Independently (on their own) – the antibodies work with the body's immune system to kill cancer cells in the same way infections are destroyed. They can directly cause cancer cells to die or stimulate the immune system to kill them:

- Antibodies that bind to an antigen called CD20 on the surface of B cells attract immune system cells to destroy the B cells they are attached to. They also help the B cells destroy themselves. These drugs include rituximab and newer anti-CD20 antibodies such as ofatumumab and obinutuzumab. These types of antibodies are used in the treatment of B-cell lymphomas, which develop when B cells become abnormal.

- Antibodies that activate the immune system to destroy abnormal cells include drugs called checkpoint inhibitors, such as nivolumab and pembrolizumab.

With chemotherapy – the antibodies cause the cancer cells to be more sensitive to the chemotherapy, making the chemotherapy work better. Many antibodies are given alongside chemotherapy as part of a regimen (combination of drugs).

Delivering other therapies – the antibody takes the other therapy directly to the lymphoma cells, allowing strong treatments to be given with fewer effects on normal cells (side effects). These treatments include:

- antibody–drug conjugates: a strong chemotherapy drug is joined to an antibody, for example brentuximab vedotin (brand name Adcetris®)
- antibody–toxin conjugates: a toxin (a naturally occurring poison) is joined to an antibody, for example the experimental drug denileukin diftitox (brand name Ontak®)
- radioimmunotherapy: a radioactive particle is joined to an antibody, for example 90Y-ibritumomab tiuxetan (Zevalin®).

Several antibody therapies are already being used to treat lymphoma, and many others are in development. Find out which antibody therapies and other targeted drugs are approved to treat your type of lymphoma on our regularly updated targeted drugs page.

Some antibody therapies are in clinical trials to test how safe and effective they are in treating certain types of lymphoma.

19 Rituximab for lymphoma

Although rituximab can be used to treat other diseases such as rheumatoid arthritis, this information is only about its use in treating lymphoma.

19.1 What is rituximab?

Rituximab was the first antibody therapy used in the treatment of lymphoma. It was designed to bind (stick) to an antigen, a protein on the surface of a cell, called 'CD20'. CD20 is found on the surface of specialised white blood cells called B lymphocytes (or B cells) that normally fight infection. Most types of lymphoma develop from a B cell. Rituximab is therefore used to treat many types of B-cell lymphoma.

Rituximab is not given to treat all types of B-cell lymphomas. The cancerous B cells need to have the CD20 protein on their surface for rituximab to be effective. This means rituximab is not given for classical Hodgkin lymphoma, as the lymphoma cells do not usually have CD20. However, rituximab is often used to treat a rare type of Hodgkin lymphoma called 'nodular lymphocyte-predominant Hodgkin lymphoma' (NLPHL), as this type of lymphoma does have CD20 on its cells.

Rituximab does not work in lymphomas that have developed from T lymphocytes (T-cell lymphomas). However, the cancerous T cells in some types of T-cell lymphoma, like angioimmunoblastic T-cell lymphoma (AITL), can cause abnormal numbers of B cells to be produced. In these cases, rituximab can be given.

Healthy B cells also have CD20 on their surface. This means rituximab destroys some healthy B cells that are not part of the lymphoma, too. As B cells are part of the immune system, you may be more likely to get infections during treatment. Your body will replace the healthy B cells when you have finished treatment with rituximab.

Several biosimilars to rituximab (medicines that are almost identical to rituximab but are made by different manufacturers) have been approved for use in Europe and are used in the UK. These are different brands of rituximab. Rituximab biosimilars are only approved for use if they are proven to work in the same way as the original rituximab, which has the brand name MabThera®.

19.2 Who can have it?

Rituximab is approved in Europe to treat adults with:

- follicular lymphoma
- diffuse large B-cell lymphoma (DLBCL)
- chronic lymphocytic leukaemia (CLL).

It is also widely used to treat other types of B-cell non-Hodgkin lymphoma and nodular lymphocyte-predominant Hodgkin lymphoma (NLPHL).

Rituximab is not currently approved to treat under 18s with lymphoma, but clinical trials have confirmed benefit in some types of childhood lymphoma such as diffuse large B-cell lymphoma (DLBCL). It is used routinely in this condition.

19.2.1 Is it available on the NHS in the UK?

Rituximab is widely available on the NHS throughout the UK to treat B-cell non-Hodgkin lymphomas, in addition to CLL and NLPHL.

19.3 Benefits

Rituximab works in many types of lymphoma, either alone or combined with chemotherapy. It is most often given together with chemotherapy as a chemo-immunotherapy regimen (combination of drugs).

If you have a B-cell non-Hodgkin lymphoma, CLL or NLPHL, you are likely to have chemo-immunotherapy as your first treatment. The choice of chemotherapy that is given with rituximab depends on what type of lymphoma you have and your individual circumstances. There are now different antibodies that work on the same target as rituximab – a protein called CD20 – and some people have those as part of their chemo-immunotherapy regimen instead of rituximab.

Rituximab usually causes fewer side effects than chemotherapy, so it is sometimes used on its own for people who are not well enough to be treated with chemotherapy.

Some people with advanced-stage follicular lymphoma that is not yet causing problems might be offered a short course of rituximab to delay the need for more treatment.

In some types of lymphoma, such as follicular lymphoma and mantle cell lymphoma, rituximab is also used as maintenance therapy after chemotherapy has been completed. For maintenance, rituximab is given on its own once every 2 to 3 months, usually for around 2 years. Maintenance therapy helps to keep the disease in remission (no evidence of lymphoma) by targeting and killing lymphoma cells left over after chemotherapy.

Some of the benefits of rituximab seen in clinical trials include the following:

- **Adding rituximab to chemotherapy to treat some types of high-grade lymphoma increases the chance of cure and prolongs life expectancy.** This is best demonstrated for DLBCL, where the addition of rituximab to chemotherapy has enabled many more patients to be cured of their lymphoma and live longer than they would have done without it.

- **Adding rituximab to chemotherapy to treat several types of lymphoma increases the length of remissions.** Studies in follicular lymphoma, for example, have shown that people who had rituximab added to their chemotherapy lived for around three times longer without their lymphoma getting worse than those who had chemotherapy alone. In CLL, people treated with rituximab and chemotherapy had several more months of remission before they needed more treatment compared with those treated with chemotherapy alone.

- **People who do not respond to other treatments might respond to rituximab.** In a study of people with follicular lymphoma who had not responded to previous treatment, around half had a reduction in their lymphoma when rituximab was given on its own.

- **Having maintenance rituximab for follicular lymphoma can reduce the risk of the lymphoma coming back by half.** Maintenance hasn't been shown to increase the time people live, but it means they might have a longer period before they need more treatment. Some people might never need more treatment.

- **Maintenance therapy for mantle cell lymphoma increases the time people live overall and increases the time they stay in remission.** Maintenance is usually given after initial treatment and a stem cell transplant, but might also be given after initial treatment to people who are not able to have a stem cell transplant.

- **A short course of rituximab for advanced-stage follicular lymphoma without troublesome symptoms might delay the need for more treatment.** Fewer people given a short course of rituximab need treatment after 3 years than those who had no treatment initially. Some people might never need more treatment for their lymphoma.

If your lymphoma comes back or doesn't respond to your first treatment, you might have further treatment that includes rituximab, for example it might be given with a different chemotherapy regimen.

19.4 How is it given?

Rituximab is usually given in a day-care unit. If you are having rituximab together with chemotherapy, it is usually given just before the chemotherapy drugs on the first day of each cycle. Rituximab can also be given on its own for some types of lymphoma and for some people who are not able to have chemotherapy at all.

Rituximab can also be given as a short course of treatment for follicular lymphoma to delay the need for further treatment. In these cases, rituximab is usually given once a week for 4 weeks.

Rituximab is usually given as an intravenous infusion (through a vein). Depending on your type of lymphoma, it may be given by subcutaneous injection (injection into the layer of fat just beneath the skin). You can only be given subcutaneous rituximab if you have received at least one full dose by intravenous infusion over the course of 1 day.

19.4.1 Intravenous infusion

The first infusion is given slowly, over 4 to 5 hours. Remaining doses can be given more quickly – over about an hour – if you have not had a bad reaction previously.

Your dose depends on the type of lymphoma you have. For some types of lymphoma, the dose is calculated based on your weight.

19.4.2 Subcutaneous injection

The rituximab subcutaneous injection was approved in Europe in 2014 for use in people with follicular lymphoma and DLBCL. This method may not be available at every centre and in England, the NHS only funds subcutaneous rituximab for maintenance treatment. Only certain brands of rituximab can be given by subcutaneous injection.

When given by subcutaneous injection, rituximab is injected slowly over about 5 minutes into the abdomen (tummy).

In clinical trials, the subcutaneous injection was just as effective as the intravenous infusion.

The same dose of rituximab is usually recommended for everyone treated by subcutaneous injection, regardless of body weight.

19.5 Possible side effects

All medicines can cause side effects (unwanted effects of treatment). Only the most common side effects are described on this page. Your medical team should discuss the most up-to-date information with you. Read all the information you are given about rituximab, which will tell you more about possible side effects. The best time to ask any questions you might have about possible side effects is before you start treatment.

You also need to tell your medical team about any other conditions you have and any medicines, supplements or complementary therapies you are taking before you start any new treatment.

Your medical team monitor you closely for side effects during treatment. They can tell you what to look out for and who to contact if you have any problems.

Rituximab generally doesn't cause many side effects because it targets only B cells. Some people will not have any side effects. Tell your medical team if you develop any new problems during or after rituximab treatment.

The most common side effects happen in the first 2 hours of the first infusion and are known as 'infusion-related' side effects. These include fever, chills and shivering. Although they are usually called 'infusion-related', the same side effects can happen with subcutaneous rituximab, not just the intravenous form.

Most people (nearly 8 in every 10 people) have some infusion-related side effects with their first dose. The first dose of rituximab is always given as an infusion so your reaction can be monitored and the infusion stopped or slowed down if necessary. You can only have subcutaneous rituximab if you didn't have a bad reaction to the intravenous form, because the subcutaneous form can't be stopped mid-treatment if you have a bad reaction. Infusion-related side effects are less likely to happen with later doses. The number of people with infusion-related side effects drops to below 1 in 100 people after eight doses of rituximab.

To help prevent side effects developing, you should be given medicines before your treatment starts. These include paracetamol and an antihistamine, but you might be given other medicines as well. You are closely monitored during your treatment, with your temperature, pulse and blood pressure being checked regularly. If you think you are having any side effects, tell your nurse straightaway.

The other most common side effects of rituximab, which can affect more than 1 in 10 people, are:

- infections, including bacterial infections and viral infections
- bronchitis (inflammation of the airways in the lungs), which might cause symptoms like a cough
- effects on the blood: leucopenia (low levels of white blood cells), including neutropenia (low levels of neutrophils, a type of white blood cell), febrile neutropenia (neutropenia with a fever) and thrombocytopenia (low platelets)
- swelling beneath the skin
- nausea
- skin rash, itching
- hair loss
- a feeling of weakness
- headache
- low antibody levels.

If you have troublesome side effects, rituximab may be stopped or the infusion slowed down for a while. Once the effects have eased off, it will be slowly restarted, and you will be carefully monitored.

19.5.1 Other severe side effects

Severe side effects with rituximab are very uncommon but other side effects that could be severe include:

- severe infusion-related reactions
- increased risk of infection
- other low blood counts.

Severe infusion-related reactions

A small number of people who are given rituximab have a more severe infusion-related reaction, which could be:

- **Cytokine release syndrome**: Cytokines are small proteins that are important in cell signalling. Rituximab can cause a lot of cytokines to be released at once, causing an inflammatory response throughout your whole body. You might have fever, chills, swelling and difficulty breathing, which usually start between 30 minutes and 2 hours after treatment begins.

- **Tumour lysis syndrome**: When rituximab kills cancer cells, they release chemicals as they break down. If a lot of cells break down at once, this can cause problems for your kidneys. Tumour lysis syndrome is rare. It is more likely to occur when you have a lot of lymphoma in your body or a large number of cancerous cells circulating in your blood. It is most likely to happen in people with CLL. If your doctor thinks you could be affected, you might be given medication to prevent this before treatment. Rituximab might also be administered more slowly than usual or over 2 days. You will be monitored carefully.

- **Anaphylactic allergic or hypersensitivity reaction**: Some people have allergic reactions to rituximab or one of the components of the drug solution. These tend to happen within a few minutes of the drug being started. Symptoms are similar to those for cytokine release syndrome.

If you have any of these reactions, treatment will be stopped straightaway. You will be given drugs to treat the symptoms and lessen the reaction, but you might need to stay in hospital to be monitored to make sure you are recovering well. Sometimes the drug can be carefully restarted when you have recovered.

Increased risk of infection
Rituximab, especially if given with chemotherapy, can lower the number of specialised white blood cells (neutrophils) available to fight infections. When you don't have enough neutrophils, you have neutropenia. As it targets B cells, rituximab can also damage healthy B cells that are part of your body's defence against infection.

Until your white blood cell counts recover, you have a higher chance of getting an infection. You should tell your medical team immediately if you develop any sign of infection, such as a temperature, cough, diarrhoea, pain when passing urine, or if you feel generally unwell.

A very small number of people receiving rituximab develop a viral brain infection known as progressive multifocal leukoencephalopathy (PML). This is a serious complication but fortunately it is very rare.

Other low blood counts
Red blood cell and platelet counts can drop after treatment with rituximab, especially if you are having chemotherapy too. A lack of red blood cells (anaemia) can make you feel

tired and short of breath. A lack of platelets (thrombocytopenia) makes you more likely to bleed or bruise easily.

19.5.2 Are there any side effects with rituximab by subcutaneous injection?

The same side effects occur with subcutaneous rituximab as with intravenous rituximab. However, if you are treated with subcutaneous rituximab you might have a reaction around the area where you had the injection. This can include pain, swelling and rash. These normally go away without treatment.

19.6 Precautions

Your doctor may reduce your dose and monitor you more closely or recommend that you do not take rituximab if you have certain other conditions. For example, people who have had certain infections in the past, such as hepatitis B, need to be monitored carefully to make sure the infection doesn't flare up during treatment with rituximab.

Make sure you tell your doctor about any medical conditions and any medicines you are taking.

Your doctor might also change your dose if you experience troublesome side effects.

Rituximab has not been approved for use in people under 18.

Rituximab is not recommended for pregnant or breastfeeding women. Women should use effective contraception to prevent pregnancy during treatment and for 12 months afterwards. If you are pregnant and need treatment, your doctor will discuss the risks and benefits of all the possible treatments with you. There is no evidence that rituximab affects your fertility. Do not breastfeed if you are being treated with rituximab or for 12 months after your treatment has finished.

You should not be immunised with live vaccines while you are receiving treatment with an antibody or for at least 6 months afterwards. Some doctors recommend that you avoid live vaccines for longer so it is important to discuss this with your doctor. Live vaccines are given for rubella, mumps and measles (often given together as the MMR), shingles, tuberculosis and yellow fever. The nasal spray flu vaccine is also a live vaccine, but the injection is not. You can still have other non-live vaccines, such as the winter flu jab. However, these might not be as effective as usual.

Research has shown that immunisations you had in the past, such as MMR, should still be effective after treatment with rituximab.

20 Newer antibodies against

20.1 Antibodies targeting CD20

All cells have different antigens (proteins) on their surface. CD20 is a protein on B cells (the white blood cells that are abnormal in B-cell lymphomas).

Antibodies bind (stick) to antigens on cells so your immune system can recognise and destroy the cell the antibody is attached to. Antibodies are produced naturally by your body to fight infection. Antibody treatments are made in a laboratory and are designed to bind a specific target on a cell.

Rituximab was the first antibody targeting CD20 to be approved to treat people with lymphoma. It allows your immune system to target cells it is bound to, including lymphoma cells. Your body can then get rid of the targeted cells. Rituximab is now used as part of treatment for many people with lymphoma.

There are newer antibodies that, like rituximab, target the CD20 antigen. Because CD20 is only on B cells, these are mainly used to treat B-cell lymphomas.

There are two newer antibodies targeting CD20 that are already approved for some people with lymphoma:

- ofatumumab
- obinutuzumab.

20.2 Ofatumumab (Arzerra®)

Ofatumumab is an antibody that binds to a slightly different part of CD20 to rituximab. It also binds to CD20 for longer than rituximab.

20.2.1 Who can have it?

At the time of writing, ofatumumab is only approved in Europe for chronic lymphocytic leukaemia (CLL). It might be available for other types of lymphoma in clinical trials.

Ofatumumab can be used for:

- People with CLL who are having treatment for the first time and who can't have fludarabine (a chemotherapy drug often used as part of the first treatment for CLL). Ofatumumab is given with chlorambucil or bendamustine chemotherapy.

- People with CLL that has relapsed (come back). It is given with the chemotherapy drugs fludarabine and cyclophosphamide.
- People whose CLL did not respond ('refractory') to previous treatments with fludarabine and alemtuzumab (another targeted drug). Ofatumumab is given on its own in this case.

Is it available on the NHS in the UK?

You might be able to have ofatumumab on the NHS if you are having your first treatment for CLL and you can't have fludarabine or bendamustine, for example because you have other health conditions that mean it would be unsafe for you to have them.

You won't be able to have ofatumumab on the NHS if you have already had treatment for your CLL. It has been assessed for refractory CLL, but it is not funded for this use in the UK.

20.2.2 Benefits

For first-line treatment of CLL, ofatumumab was tested in a major clinical trial of 447 people who had not yet had treatment for their CLL but who couldn't have fludarabine. In the trial, some people were given chlorambucil chemotherapy alone and others were given chlorambucil with ofatumumab. The people who had ofatumumab and chlorambucil lived for nearly twice as long without their CLL getting worse than those who just had chlorambucil (22 months compared with 13 months).

Ofatumumab was tested in a clinical trial of 223 people who had previously had fludarabine or alemtuzumab and had not responded to treatment. Ofatumumab was not compared with another treatment in this trial. Half of the people who had ofatumumab responded to the treatment.

Ofatumumab has also been tested in clinical trials for people who have had other treatments but whose CLL **has** come back. It may increase the time it takes for CLL to get worse in these people.

20.2.3 How is it given?

Ofatumumab is given intravenously (into a vein). It can take several hours to have a dose of ofatumumab.

For the first dose, you have only a small amount of ofatumumab. You start the treatment at a low rate of infusion (how quickly it is given into your vein) that is increased gradually. These precautions allow your medical team to see how the treatment affects you and manage any side effects. You also have other treatments like paracetamol, antihistamines (anti-allergy drugs) and steroids to help prevent side effects. If you do have problems, the infusion might be slowed down again, or stopped.

If you don't have troublesome side effects, you have your first full dose a week later.

If it is part of your first treatment for CLL, you then have ofatumumab monthly for up to 11 more doses.

20.2.4 Possible side effects

All medicines can cause side effects (unwanted effects of treatment). As ofatumumab is a new treatment, more information about possible side effects is still being gathered.

Ofatumumab can cause infusion-related side effects (effects that occur while the treatment is given or shortly afterwards), such as shivers, fevers, headache and other flu-like symptoms. Severe reactions can occur. They can make you feel very ill. If you have a severe reaction, you have treatment to manage the symptoms and ofatumumab might be stopped until you are better. These infusion reactions are more common with your first infusion, which is why the first dose is given slowly and at a low dose. The other medicines you have before and during your ofatumumab infusion help to reduce your risk of severe infusion reactions.

Other common side effects (effects that occur in more than 1 in every 10 people) include:

- increased risk of infection (including colds, sore throat and pneumonia)
- neutropenia (a drop in the number of neutrophils in your blood. Neutrophils are a type of white blood cell that fights infection – neutropenia can increase your risk of infection)
- anaemia (shortage of red blood cells)
- nausea (feeling sick) and diarrhoea (loose stools)
- fever (high temperature)
- rash
- difficulty breathing and cough
- fatigue (extreme tiredness).

Serious complications are not common but could include:

- tumour lysis syndrome (complications caused by the rapid breakdown of lymphoma cells)
- bowel obstruction (blockage)

- very rarely, progressive multifocal leukoencephalopathy (PML), which is a viral brain infection.

This is not a complete list of side effects that have been reported. Ask your medical team for the most up-to-date information about possible side effects. Ask all the questions you have. You also need to tell your medical team about any other conditions you have and any medicines, supplements or complementary therapies you are taking before you start any new treatment.

20.2.5 Are there any other precautions?

As ofatumumab reduces the number of B cells in your body, it can affect your response to vaccinations. You should not have any live vaccines (for example, the shingles vaccine) during your treatment and after treatment until the number of B cells in your blood has returned to normal. Talk to your doctor about the risks and benefits of any other vaccinations before you have them.

If you've ever had hepatitis B (an infection of your liver), you might need antiviral treatment to prevent the infection flaring up while you are having ofatumumab. If you have active hepatitis B, you won't be able to have ofatumumab until it is under control.

You need to be monitored closely if you have heart problems. You might need to have tests to see how well your heart is working before you start treatment.

People who are pregnant should not usually have ofatumumab during their pregnancy in case it could harm the unborn baby. You must use contraception to prevent pregnancy for at least 12 months after treatment and you must not breastfeed for the same period.

20.3 Obinutuzumab (Gazyvaro®)

Obinutuzumab is an antibody that has been modified to bind more tightly to CD20 than rituximab. It was previously known as GA101.

20.3.1 Who can have it?

At the time of writing, obinutuzumab is only approved in Europe for chronic lymphocytic leukaemia and follicular lymphoma. It might be available for other types of lymphoma in clinical trials.

Chronic lymphocytic leukaemia (CLL)

Obinutuzumab can be used for:

- People who need their first treatment for CLL and who can't have fludarabine (a type of chemotherapy often used as part of the first treatment for CLL). It is given with chlorambucil chemotherapy.

Follicular lymphoma

Obinutuzumab can be used for:

- People who need their first treatment for advanced-stage follicular lymphoma. It is given with chemotherapy and followed by obinutuzumab maintenance.
- People whose lymphoma was refractory (didn't respond) to treatment containing rituximab or whose lymphoma got worse during or within 6 months after treatment containing rituximab. It is given with bendamustine chemotherapy.

Is it available on the NHS?

Some people with CLL and follicular lymphoma might be able to have obinutuzumab as part of their treatment on the NHS.

20.3.1.1.1 CLL

You might be able to have obinutuzumab with chlorambucil on the NHS as a first treatment for CLL if you can't have fludarabine or bendamustine.

Follicular lymphoma

You can only have obinutuzumab on the NHS as part of your first treatment for follicular lymphoma if you have risk factors that mean your lymphoma is at moderate or high risk of getting worse soon after treatment. This is because evidence from clinical trials showed that people with these risk factors are more likely to benefit from having obinutuzumab instead of the usual treatment of rituximab with their chemotherapy. People in Scotland can't currently have obinutuzumab as part of their first treatment as it has not been recommended by the Scottish Medicines Consortium (SMC).

If you previously had rituximab as part of your treatment and your lymphoma did not respond or got worse within 6 months, you might be able to have obinutuzumab with bendamustine in some parts of the UK. In England, it is available on the NHS through the Cancer Drugs Fund. In Scotland, it is available routinely on the NHS.

20.3.2 Benefits

Clinical trials have shown that obinutuzumab could be more effective than rituximab for some people.

CLL

Clinical trials have been done in people with CLL who had other health conditions that meant they couldn't have fludarabine. The results showed that adding obinutuzumab to chlorambucil more than doubled the time people lived without their CLL getting worse compared with chlorambucil alone. Obinutuzumab with chlorambucil also significantly improved outcomes compared with rituximab with chlorambucil.

Follicular lymphoma

For people with untreated advanced-stage follicular lymphoma, obinutuzumab with chemotherapy slightly increases the time people live without their lymphoma getting worse compared with rituximab and chemotherapy. However, the new combination can cause more side effects. People with higher-risk untreated follicular lymphoma might particularly benefit from having obinutuzumab instead of rituximab.

Adding obinutuzumab to bendamustine chemotherapy for people with follicular lymphoma that has relapsed shortly after having rituximab or didn't respond to rituximab significantly improves outcomes. People having obinutuzumab with bendamustine live, on average, more than twice as long without their lymphoma getting worse than those who have bendamustine alone.

20.3.3 How is it given?

Obinutuzumab is given intravenously (into a vein). It takes several hours to have each dose.

CLL

For CLL, obinutuzumab is given slowly to begin with. You have a small amount of the drug at first and it is given at a slow infusion rate (how quickly it is given into your vein). You have the rest of the dose later the same day or the following day. The infusion rate may be increased gradually. You are closely monitored for side effects. If you do have problems, the infusion might be slowed down again, or stopped.

You have obinutuzumab twice more in the first month. You then have obinutuzumab once every 4 weeks. Each 4-week period is a cycle of treatment. You can have up to 6 cycles in total.

Follicular lymphoma

For follicular lymphoma, you have obinutuzumab once a week for 3 weeks. You then have obinutuzumab once every 3 or 4 weeks, depending on what chemotherapy you are having with it. You can have 6 to 8 cycles of obinutuzumab.

If you have follicular lymphoma and you responded to treatment with obinutuzumab, you might then have maintenance therapy. Maintenance therapy is given after initial treatment has put the lymphoma into remission (no evidence of lymphoma on scans). It aims to make your remission last longer. For maintenance, obinutuzumab is given every 2 months for up to 2 years.

20.3.4 Possible side effects

All medicines can cause side effects (unwanted effects of treatment). As obinutuzumab is a new treatment, more information about possible side effects is still being gathered.

Obinutuzumab can cause infusion-related side effects (effects that occur while the treatment is given or shortly afterwards), such as shivers, fevers, headache and other flu-like symptoms. Severe reactions can occur. They can make you feel very ill. If you have a severe reaction, you have treatment to manage the symptoms and ofatumumab might be stopped until you are better. Infusion reactions are more common with your first infusion, which is why the first dose is given slowly and at a low dose. You are given other medicines (for example, paracetamol and antihistamines) before and during the obinutuzumab infusion to reduce your risk of severe infusion reactions.

Other common side effects (effects that occur in more than 1 in every 10 people) of obinutuzumab include:

- increased risk of infection (for example colds, sore throats, pneumonia, urinary tract infections, cold sores)
- neutropenia (a drop in the number of neutrophils you have, a type of white blood cell) and leucopenia (low white blood cells of different types)
- increased risk of bruising and bleeding because of thrombocytopenia (low platelets)
- anaemia (low red blood cells)
- cough
- joint pain

- headache
- fever
- weakness
- difficulty sleeping
- hair loss
- itching
- diarrhoea or constipation.

Serious complications are not common but could include:

- tumour lysis syndrome (complications caused by the rapid breakdown of cancer cells)
- severe infections
- worsening of existing heart conditions
- very rarely, progressive multifocal leukoencephalopathy (PML), which is a viral brain infection.

This is not a complete list of side effects that have been reported. Ask your medical team for the most up-to-date information about possible side effects. Ask all the questions you have. You also need to tell your medical team about any other conditions you have and any medicines, supplements or complementary therapies you are taking before you start any new treatment.

20.3.5 Are there any other precautions?

As ofatumumab reduces the number of B cells in your body, it can affect your response to vaccinations. You should not have any live vaccines (for example, the shingles vaccine) during your treatment and after treatment until the number of B cells in your blood has returned to normal. Talk to your doctor about the risks and benefits of any other vaccinations before you have them.

If you've ever had hepatitis B (an infection of your liver), you might need antiviral treatment to prevent it flaring up while you are having ofatumumab. If you have active hepatitis B, you won't be able to have obinutuzumab until it is under control.

You need to be monitored closely if you have heart problems. You might need to have tests to see how well your heart is working before you start treatment.

People who are pregnant should not usually have obinutuzumab during their pregnancy in case it could harm the unborn baby. You should use contraception to prevent pregnancy for at least 18 months after treatment and you must not breastfeed for the same period.

21 Targeted drugs for lymphoma

21.1 What are targeted drugs?

Targeted drugs are being used more and more for people with lymphoma.

There are lots of different names for targeted drugs. You might hear them called 'targeted therapies', 'biological therapies' or 'immunotherapies'.

Your whole body is made up of lots of different types of cells that do different jobs. Lymphoma develops when a type of white blood cell that fights infection (a lymphocyte) doesn't work properly and these abnormal cells start to build up in your body. Scientists are continually finding out more about the changes that cause cells to go out of control, resulting in lymphoma. This research helps them to find drugs that work on the abnormal cells.

Targeted treatments affect processes in cells. They work in different ways to stop cancer cells growing or dividing, to cause cancer cells to die or to use your own immune system to help your body get rid of cancer cells. Targeted drugs work on lymphoma cells more precisely than chemotherapy, reducing the effect of treatment on healthy cells. This aims to reduce the side effects of treatment, as well as making it more effective.

Rituximab was the first targeted immunotherapy drug used to treat lymphoma. There are now biosimilars to rituximab, which are new drugs designed to be essentially the same as rituximab and to work in the same way. Many other targeted drugs are now being used for people with lymphoma, some in routine use and many others in clinical trials (research studies that test medical treatments in people).

21.2 Who can have targeted drugs?

Before they can be used routinely, targeted drugs are tested in clinical trials to make sure they are safe and to see how effective they are at treating lymphoma. Clinical trials also help doctors find out who would benefit from the treatment and if the new treatment is better than the treatment that is usually used.

Some targeted drugs, like rituximab, are already used for lots of people with lymphoma. Others are used for a few people in specific situations, often for:

- people who have been treated before but need more treatment because their lymphoma has relapsed (come back)

- people who didn't respond well to their previous treatment (refractory lymphoma)
- people who can't have other standard treatments.

Some targeted drugs are starting to be used as a first treatment (first-line) for people with some types of lymphoma.

The following section summarises which drugs are currently approved for people with lymphoma in the UK. You might want to read only about the treatments for the type of lymphoma you have. We have more detailed information about many of these drugs.

Note that the drugs described on this page are newer treatments, so information about the possible side effects, including late effects (side effects that can occur months or years after treatment is finished), is still being gathered. Your team should discuss the most up-to-date information with you if you are going to be treated with any of these drugs.

21.3 What targeted drugs are approved for lymphoma?

Different types of targeted therapies work in different ways. You might hear them called by their drug name or their brand name (the pharmaceutical company's name for them, which is given in brackets in the list below).

Types of targeted therapies approved for use in people with lymphoma in Europe include:

- antibody treatments, for example rituximab, ofatumumab (Arzerra®) and obinutuzumab (Gazyvaro®)

- combined treatments that use antibodies to deliver chemotherapy or radiotherapy to lymphoma cells, for example brentuximab vedotin (Adcetris®) and Zevalin® (90Y-ibritumomab tiuxetan)
- drugs that block signals or the function of certain proteins within the lymphoma cells, which, depending how they work, can be grouped as:
  - cell signal blockers, for example ibrutinib (Imbruvica®), idelalisib (Zydelig®) and temsirolimus (Torisel®)
  - proteasome inhibitors, for example bortezomib (Velcade®)
  - immunomodulators, which change how your immune system works, for example lenalidomide (Revlimid®)
- programmed cell death inducers, which block proteins that keep lymphoma cells alive, for example venetoclax (Venclyxto™)
- checkpoint inhibitors, which allow the immune system to recognise and kill lymphoma cells, for example nivolumab (Opdivo®) and pembrolizumab (Keytruda®)
- CAR T-cells, where your own T cells (a type of white blood cell that fights infection) are genetically modified to help your immune system recognise and kill lymphoma cells, for example axicabtagene clioleucel (Yescarta®) and tisagenlecleucel (Kymriah®).

The following alphabetical list shows what drugs are currently approved for different types of lymphoma. Find out more about the drugs by following the links.

If your type of lymphoma is not below, then there were no targeted drugs approved to treat your type of lymphoma at the time of writing. Visit our clinical trial database, Lymphoma TrialsLink, to see if there are any trials researching targeted drugs for your type of lymphoma.

21.4 Lymphoma research and drugs in development

Drug development is a long process. New drugs have to undergo rigorous tests to demonstrate that their potential benefits outweigh their potential risks before they can be approved. Many of the drugs in clinical trials do not show enough benefit to undergo further testing.

There are many other ways to target lymphoma cells and scientists are developing and testing drugs that work in different ways to those already described.

22 Lymphoma drug development, approval and funding

why drug development takes so long, why drugs are so expensive and how you can find out whether a drug might be funded on the NHS.

22.1 Drug development

There is much excitement about new, targeted drugs for people with lymphoma, but drug development and approval is a long and expensive process. It can be frustrating hearing about new drugs that could improve outcomes for people with lymphoma when these are not yet available to you.

The time and cost to develop a drug varies hugely but on average, it takes around 12.5 years for a large pharmaceutical company to develop a drug from discovery to approval and costs around £1.15 billion. Thousands of drugs are tested for use in lymphoma treatment, but out of those, only very few are safe and effective in treating lymphoma and are approved. Although many won't be approved, results from tests with these drugs are very useful in informing future tests and drug development. This process means that pharmaceutical companies have a lot of costs to cover, and is one reason why new drugs can be very expensive.

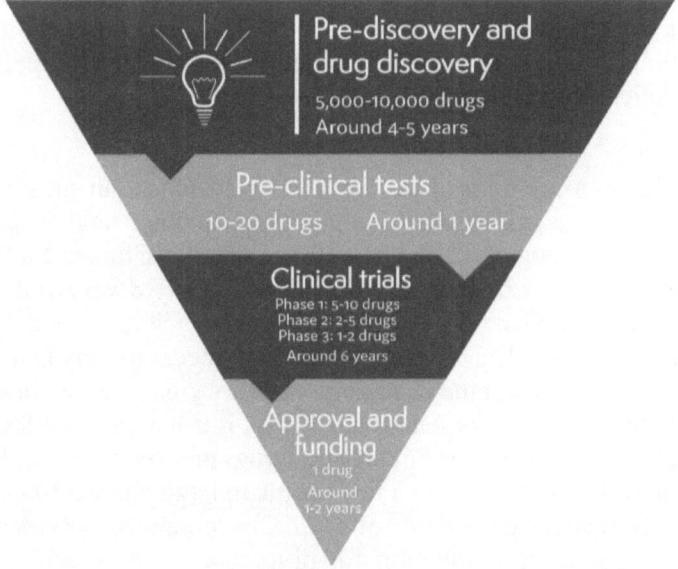

Figure: The drug development process for drugs in general

22.1.1 Pre-discovery and drug discovery

The first stage in drug development involves research to understand a disease. This research underpins the search for possible drugs – it helps to identify targets for a drug to act on. Researchers then search for drugs that act on the targets they've identified. Thousands of possible drugs are tested in this way for each drug that eventually becomes approved for use in people.

22.1.2 Pre-clinical tests

Before a drug can be tested in humans, it undergoes extensive testing in laboratories and on animals. These tests help find out how the drug works, what effects it might have in the body, and what dosage should be safe to start with in clinical trials. If serious problems are detected in pre-clinical tests, a drug won't be tested in people.

22.1.3 Clinical trials

Although pre-clinical testing gives researchers an idea of how a drug might affect people, these findings have to be tested thoroughly in people with the disease. Clinical trials are where the drug is tested in people. Only a very small proportion of the drugs identified in research are tested in clinical trials. The clinical trial testing process usually takes several years, but the exact time can vary greatly depending on the drug and the health conditions it is being tested for. Clinical trials are done in phases. Drugs proceed from small phase 1 trials involving a few people to large phase 3 trials, often involving hundreds of people, as more is learnt about them. It is very common for drugs not to show enough benefit in early phase trials for their development to continue. Cancer drugs often start out being tested in lots of different types of cancer, and are eventually only tested in the types of cancer in which they are most effective.

Visit Lymphoma TrialsLink .

The next sections explain what happens if a drug shows benefits in clinical trials and the pharmaceutical company apply for it to be approved.

22.2 Drug approval

Your doctor can only give you treatments that are approved for use in Europe (unless you are in a clinical trial).

The approval process is designed to keep you safe and to make sure you only have treatments that are likely to benefit you.

Being approved is not the same as being funded on the NHS. When a drug is approved, it is assessed by funding bodies in the UK to decide whether the benefits of the drug are worth its costs.

22.2.1 Who approves new drugs?

If clinical trials show that a new drug significantly improves outcomes for people with lymphoma, the pharmaceutical company that produced the drug applies for it to be licensed (approved) for use.

The drug company has to apply to different authorities in different parts of the world. For example:

- the Food and Drug Administration (FDA) approves drugs in the US
- the European Medicines Agency (EMA) assesses applications and recommends whether drugs should be

licensed in Europe; the European Commission (EC) then makes a decision.

At the time of writing, it is not certain how Brexit (the UK's decision to leave the European Union) will affect this process.

22.3 Funding

Once a drug has been approved in Europe, national authorities need to assess it to decide if it should be funded in each country.

In the UK, health and technology assessment bodies decide whether to make drugs available on the NHS. These are:

- the National Institute for Health and Care Excellence (NICE), whose guidance is followed in England and Wales, and often in Northern Ireland if agreed by the Department of Health, Social Services and Public Safety
- the Scottish Medicines Consortium (SMC)
- the All Wales Medicine Strategy Group (AWMSG), which looks at some drugs before a decision is reached by NICE.

22.3.1 How can I find out if a drug is available for me?

Different ways of funding cancer drugs apply in each part of the UK, so it is important that you look at the right information. The websites for each of the health and technology assessment bodies have up-to-date information on which drugs are recommended and which are currently being assessed. If the drug is still being assessed, these sites often give a date that a decision is expected. Search for your type of lymphoma or a drug name using the links below.

- If you live in England or Northern Ireland, visit the NICE website.

- If you live in Scotland, visit the SMC website.
- If you live in Wales, visit the NICE website but if a drug is not yet available, the AWSMG sometimes makes it available earlier than NICE, so you can check there too.

Our news section reports regularly on drug approvals and NICE decisions.

Funding for new drugs can change very quickly as more is learnt about the risks and benefits of each drug.

Some drugs are funded in England through schemes that give access to new drugs for a limited time while more evidence is being gathered about them. These schemes include the Cancer Drugs Fund (CDF) and the Early Access to Medicines Scheme (EAMS).

Remember to talk to your own consultant about drug availability. Even if a drug has been approved for use in your type of lymphoma, it might not be suitable for you. Some drugs might not be recommended if you have other medical conditions or are taking certain other medicines, as the drugs may interact with each other.

22.3.2 What is the Cancer Drugs Fund?

The Cancer Drugs Fund (CDF) is a source of funds that allows access to cancer drugs that are not routinely funded on the NHS. It is managed by NHS England.

In England, NICE sometimes recommends that drugs should not be available routinely on the NHS but should be made available through the CDF.

All drugs are assessed by NICE first, who decide:

- to recommend drugs for funding on the NHS
- not to recommend drugs for funding on the NHS

- to recommend drugs for funding through the CDF until more evidence is available.

If NICE decide to put a drug on the CDF list, the drug is funded through the CDF for a limited time while the drug company gathers further evidence. The drug is then assessed by NICE again to decide if it should be funded routinely on the NHS.

There is a central list of drugs available on the CDF, which details who might be able to get funding. The list is regularly updated and drugs can be added or removed.

There are currently no similar funds in Scotland, Wales or Northern Ireland. However, in those countries your doctor may be able to make an individual funding request in exceptional cases if the treatment is not routinely available on the NHS. You should discuss this with your doctor if you think that this applies to you.

22.3.3 What is the Early Access to Medicines Scheme?

The Early Access to Medicines Scheme (EAMS) is run by the UK Medicines and Healthcare Products Regulatory Agency (MHRA). This is a Government organisation that is responsible for making sure that medicines and medical devices used in the UK work well and are acceptably safe.

The MHRA can assess promising new medicines with the aim of making them available to people with no other treatment options before they are licensed in Europe. There are only a few drugs on the EAMS list at any time, but drugs for people with lymphoma sometimes appear on the list.

The MHRA assesses the available evidence to decide whether the benefits of the drug are likely to outweigh the risks. As the drugs in the scheme are new, researchers are continuing to find out more about their safety and how well they work and these are still experimental treatments until they are licensed. Once they are licensed, drugs are no longer available through EAMS.

EAMS drugs are funded in England. They may be available through drug company access schemes or through individual funding requests in other parts of the UK. If you are eligible for a drug that is on the EAMS list, you and your doctor can look at the evidence together to decide if the drug is suitable for your situation.

22.3.4 How can I access drugs that are not funded?

If a drug is approved for your type of lymphoma but is not funded in the UK, you will need to organise funding from alternative sources. Macmillan have further information on what you can do if you and your doctor think you would benefit from a drug that is not available on the NHS.

23 Brentuximab vedotin

brentuximab vedotin, a targeted drug used in the treatment of certain types of lymphoma.

23.1 What is brentuximab vedotin?

Brentuximab vedotin (Adcetris®) is an antibody-drug conjugate. This type of targeted treatment consists of an antibody joined to a chemotherapy drug. Brentuximab vedotin includes:

- a CD30 monoclonal antibody – an antibody that binds (sticks) to a protein called 'CD30', which is found on the abnormal cells in some types of lymphoma

- the chemotherapy drug monomethyl auristatin E (MMAE).

  The antibody binds (sticks) to lymphoma cells that have the CD30 protein, delivering the chemotherapy directly to the lymphoma cells.

  The chemotherapy drugs used in this type of treatment are good at killing lymphoma cells but can't be given into the bloodstream on their own because they are too toxic.

23.2 Who can have it?

Brentuximab vedotin is approved in Europe for three types of lymphoma – classical Hodgkin lymphoma, systemic anaplastic large cell lymphoma and cutaneous (skin) T-cell lymphoma. This treatment can only be used if your lymphoma cells have the CD30 protein. Cells from your biopsy sample might be tested for CD30 before you can have brentuximab vedotin.

Classical Hodgkin lymphoma

- For people whose lymphoma has relapsed (come back) after an autologous stem cell transplant (using their own stem cells), or who didn't respond to a stem cell transplant.
- For people who are not able to have a stem cell transplant or a combination of chemotherapy drugs and have had at least two other types of treatment.
- For people at high risk of their lymphoma coming back or getting worse after an autologous stem cell transplant.

Systemic anaplastic large cell lymphoma (ALCL)

- For people whose lymphoma has relapsed or has not responded to previous treatment.

Cutaneous (skin) T-cell lymphoma (CTCL)

- For people who have already received at least one other course of systemic (whole-body) drug treatment.

Brentuximab vedotin is still being tested in further clinical trials in people with these types of lymphoma, for example as a first-line treatment and in combination with other treatments. It is also being tested in other types of lymphoma. Use our searchable database to see if there's a clinical trial that might be suitable for you at Lymphoma TrialsLink.

23.2.1 Is it available on the NHS in the UK?

Brentuximab vedotin has been assessed by health authorities for some uses on the NHS in the UK. Its availability on the NHS may vary for different parts of the UK.

In Scotland

- For people with relapsed or refractory classical Hodgkin lymphoma who have had an autologous stem cell transplant, or who are not able to have a stem cell transplant or a combination of chemotherapy drugs and have had at least two other types of treatment.

In England and Wales

- For people with relapsed or refractory classical Hodgkin lymphoma who have already had a self (autologous) stem cell transplant using their own stem cells. Brentuximab vedotin is also available for people who are not able to have a stem cell transplant or a combination of chemotherapy drugs and have had at least two other types of treatment.
- For people with relapsed or refractory ALCL who are well enough for this treatment.

Brentuximab vedotin is also being assessed for other uses, for example in combination with different treatments for certain types of lymphoma. It is not currently funded for CTCL.

Northern Ireland usually follows NICE recommendations.

23.2.2 What can I do if brentuximab vedotin isn't funded for me?

If brentuximab vedotin is approved for use in your situation but isn't currently funded by the NHS, your doctor may be able to make an individual funding request in exceptional cases. Discuss this with your doctor if you think that this might apply to you.

If you have private medical insurance, ask your provider if you are covered for treatment with brentuximab vedotin.

Some people might be able to enter a clinical trial of brentuximab vedotin.

23.3 Benefits

The main trials that led to approval of brentuximab vedotin are briefly described below.

23.3.1 Benefits in classical Hodgkin lymphoma

Many people with Hodgkin lymphoma are treated successfully with their first course (line) of treatment. Sometimes, classical Hodgkin lymphoma can be difficult to treat and may need more chemotherapy (second line, or salvage treatment) and an autologous stem cell transplant. There are few treatment options if classical Hodgkin lymphoma relapses again or does not respond to a stem cell transplant. The main study in this area showed that three-quarters of 102 people treated with brentuximab vedotin responded to the treatment (their lymphoma shrank or disappeared – a partial or complete remission, respectively).

People who have had at least two other courses (lines) of treatment but are not suitable for a stem cell transplant or chemotherapy with a combination of drugs might also benefit from brentuximab vedotin. In a study of 40 people with classical Hodgkin lymphoma, just over half responded to brentuximab vedotin.

Brentuximab vedotin could also help to keep classical Hodgkin lymphoma under control for longer in people who have had a stem cell transplant but who are at high risk of their lymphoma coming back. In a study of 329 people, lymphoma stayed under control for nearly twice as long in people treated with brentuximab vedotin compared with people who received a placebo (dummy treatment).

23.3.2 Benefits in systemic ALCL

ALCL can be difficult to treat if it comes back or doesn't respond to treatment. In a study of 58 people with relapsed or refractory ALCL, 50 people responded to treatment with brentuximab vedotin.

23.3.3 Benefits in CTCL

CTCL is rare and usually requires a range of different treatments during the course of the disease. In a trial of 128 people with relapsed or refractory CTCL, more than half of people responded to treatment with brentuximab vedotin, compared with around 1 in 10 of those given other treatments.

23.4 How is it given?

You have brentuximab vedotin as an intravenous infusion (into a vein) over 30 minutes. You usually have the treatment once every 3 weeks, where each 3-week period is a 'cycle' of treatment. Most people can have the treatment in hospital as an outpatient, but some people might need to stay overnight for monitoring. On average, a response to brentuximab vedotin is seen after 4 or 5 cycles of treatment. The number of cycles of brentuximab vedotin you have depends on how you respond, how the treatment affects you and whether or not you go on to have a stem cell transplant. If brentuximab vedotin is controlling your lymphoma, you can have up to 16 cycles (1 year) of treatment. If your lymphoma stops responding or you develop side effects, you might stop treatment earlier.

23.5 Possible side effects

All medicines can cause side effects (unwanted effects of treatment). As brentuximab vedotin is a new treatment, more information about possible side effects is still being gathered.

The most common side effects of brentuximab vedotin, which can affect more than 1 in 10 people, are:

- infusion-related reactions (occurring while the treatment is given or shortly afterwards) such as shivers, fevers, and other flu-like symptoms
- gastrointestinal problems, such as nausea and vomiting, diarrhoea or constipation, abdominal (tummy) pain and weight loss
- fatigue (extreme tiredness)

- itching and rashes
- hair loss
- muscle and joint pain
- peripheral neuropathy (nerve damage that can cause problems such as pins and needles)
- infections (for example colds) and neutropenia (a drop in the number of neutrophils you have, a type of white blood cell that fights infection)
- cough and shortness of breath.

Serious complications are less common but could include:

- serious infections like pneumonia and, very rarely, progressive multifocal leukoencephalopathy (a viral brain infection, which can be fatal)
- problems with the lungs or liver, or gastrointestinal complications
- tumour lysis syndrome (complications caused by the rapid breakdown of lymphoma cells)
- demyelinating polyneuropathy (a neurological disorder characterized by slowly progressive weakness and a loss of sensation in the legs and arms)
- Stevens-Johnson syndrome (a life-threatening allergic reaction affecting the skin and mucous membranes)
- pancreatitis (inflammation of the pancreas).

This is not a complete list of side effects that have been reported. Ask your medical team for the most up-to-date information about possible side effects. Ask all the questions you have. You also need to tell your medical team about any other conditions you have and any medicines, supplements or complementary therapies you are taking before you start any new treatment.

Your medical team monitor you closely for side effects during treatment. They can tell you what to look out for and who to contact if you have any problems.

23.6 Precautions

Some people will not be able to have brentuximab vedotin because they are taking other medications or have other conditions. **Make sure you tell your doctor about any medical conditions and any medicines you are taking.** Your doctor may reduce your dose and monitor you more closely or recommend that you do not take brentuximab vedotin if you have certain other conditions. These include liver problems and kidney problems. Your doctor might also change your dose if you experience troublesome side effects.

Brentuximab vedotin has not been approved for use in people under 18.

People who are pregnant should not usually have brentuximab vedotin during their pregnancy in case it could harm the unborn baby. You must use at least two effective measures of contraception to prevent pregnancy for at least 6 months after treatment and you should not breastfeed for the same period. Discuss your treatment options with your doctor if you think you might be pregnant.

24 CAR T cells

CAR T-cell therapy, a type of targeted treatment used for certain types of high-grade (fast-growing) lymphoma.

24.1 What are CAR T cells?

CAR T cells use your own immune system to try to destroy lymphoma cells.

Lymphocytes are types of white blood cell that your body produces to help you fight infection and disease, including cancer. They are part of your immune system. Lymphocytes include T lymphocytes (T cells) and B lymphocytes (B cells), and these have different roles in your immune system.

If any of your own cells become abnormal, they are normally recognised as different by T cells and destroyed by your immune system. When a cancer (such as a lymphoma) develops, it means that the immune system, for some reason, has not detected the abnormal cancerous cells or has not been able to get rid of them. Cancer cells also develop ways to prevent the immune system attacking them. For example, some cancer cells make special proteins on their surface that tell T cells not to attack them.

In CAR T-cell therapy, your own T cells are collected and genetically modified (changed) in a laboratory. These changes allow them to recognise and kill lymphoma cells that are otherwise not detected by your immune cells. The genetically modified T cells are known as 'CAR T cells'. After they have been modified, the CAR T cells are grown in the laboratory until there are enough of them to treat your lymphoma. They are then given back to you, like a blood transfusion.

24.1.1 The parts of a CAR T cell

When CAR T cells are made, a 'chimeric antigen receptor' (CAR) is joined onto your T cells by genetic engineering in a laboratory. The CAR is made up of several parts. These usually include:

- An **antigen receptor**, which is the part that is designed to attach to a specific target on cancer cells.
- **Stimulation signals** and **activation signals**, which help the CAR T cells to multiply and survive in your body.

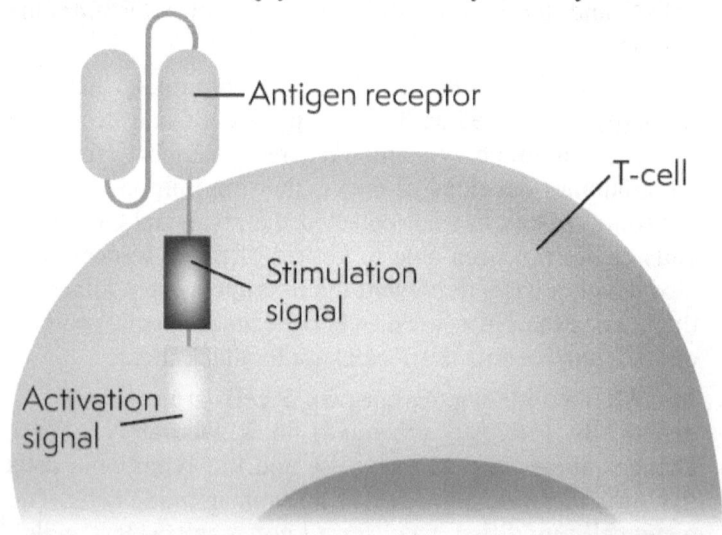

Figure: A CAR T cell

When a CAR T cell binds to a cancer cell in your body, it sends signals to tell your immune system to destroy the cell.

The various types of CAR T cell have different antigen receptors so they can target specific types of cancer cell. New CAR T cells are in development that have other parts added to them to help them survive in your body or to help switch them off if they cause problems in your body.

24.2 Who can have them?

Two types of CAR T-cell therapy are approved in Europe for some people with high-grade (fast-growing) lymphomas:

- tisagenlecleucel (Kymriah®) for some people with diffuse large B-cell lymphoma (DLBCL) who have had two or more previous courses of treatment but their lymphoma has relapsed (come back) or was refractory (did not respond to treatment)
- axicabtagene ciloleucel (Yescarta®) for some people with relapsed or refractory DLBCL or primary mediastinal large B-cell lymphoma (PMBL), who have had two or more previous courses of treatment.

Several CAR T-cell treatments are being tested in clinical trials in these and other types of lymphoma. Use our searchable database to see if there's a clinical trial that might be suitable for you at Lymphoma TrialsLink.

Note: CAR T cells are being tested and may be approved for other types of cancer, but this information is specifically about lymphoma.

24.2.1 Are they available on the NHS in the UK?

Axicabtagene ciloleucel and tisagenlecleucel are available on the NHS in England and Wales. They are not approved for use on the NHS in Scotland. At the time of writing, the Department of Health in Northern Ireland has not confirmed whether CAR T-cell therapy will be available on the NHS.

CAR T-cell therapy is a very intensive type of treatment and you have to be fit enough to have it. Even if you are suitable for this treatment and it is available to you, it is not always possible for you to have it for several reasons, for example:

- It may not be possible for your medical team to collect enough T cells from you to make the treatment.
- The laboratory might not able to successfully make the treatment.
- Your health might worsen while the treatment is being made, and you might no longer be well enough to have it.

In these cases, your specialist will consider what other treatment options are available for you.

24.3 Benefits

CAR T-cell therapy is a new type of treatment, so little is known about its long-term effects or whether any response the lymphoma has to the treatment will last long-term. Initial results from clinical trials are very encouraging, particularly for people who have few other treatment options after having standard treatments.

24.3.1 Benefits of axicabtagene ciloleucel

Around three-quarters of 101 people treated with axicabtagene ciloleucel in a clinical trial responded to treatment, with half overall having a complete response (the lymphoma was completely cleared). People who had a complete response were more likely to stay in remission (no evidence of lymphoma). The people included in the trial had DLBCL or PMBL, including DLBCL that had transformed (changed) from follicular lymphoma, double-hit or triple-hit DLBCL and people with high-grade B-cell lymphoma not otherwise specified. All of the people included in the trial had previously received treatment and their lymphoma either hadn't responded or had relapsed after at least two courses of treatment.

24.3.2 Benefits of tisagenlecleucel

Around half of 68 people treated with tisagenlecleucel in a clinical trial responded to treatment, with around a third overall having a complete response. As with axicabtagene ciloleucel, the response to tisagenlecleucel seems to be lasting in those who had a complete response. The people included in this trial all had DLBCL (including DLBCL that had transformed from follicular lymphoma) and had all received at least two previous courses of treatment.

24.4 How are they given?

CAR T-cell treatments have to be made individually for each person. This process can take several weeks. You might be able to have other treatments, such as chemotherapy, to keep your lymphoma under control while the CAR T cells are being made.

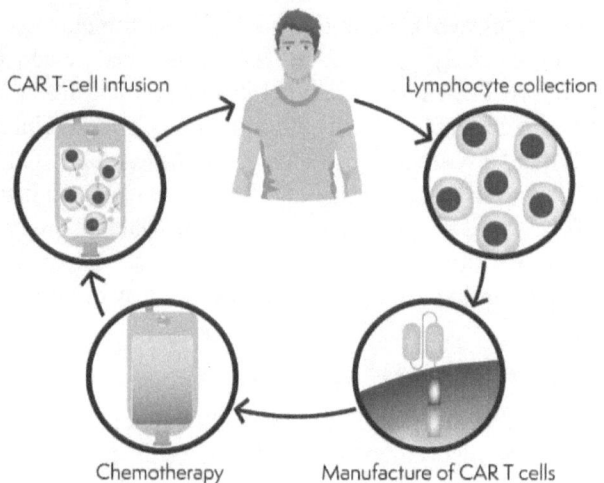

Figure: The CAR T cell treatment process

24.4.1 Step 1: Lymphocyte collection

Your lymphocytes are collected so that the T cells can be modified in the laboratory. This collection process is called 'leukapheresis'. In leukapheresis, your blood is taken from a line (thin tube) in one arm, and passed through a machine. The machine separates the lymphocytes (T cells and other types of lymphocyte) from your blood and collects them. The rest of your blood is returned to your bloodstream through another line. Only lymphocytes that are in your blood can be collected through this process, so not all of your lymphocytes are taken.

24.4.2 Step 2: Manufacture of CAR T cells

The T cells are modified and allowed to multiply in the laboratory until there are enough cells to make the treatment effective. You need lots of CAR T cells in your body so that they can survive, multiply even more and destroy most or all of the cancer cells.

Making CAR T cells is complicated and usually takes several weeks.

Your doctor needs to check that you are still well enough to have the CAR T-cell treatment when it is ready. Some people get more unwell while the CAR T-cell treatment is being made, as their lymphoma might get worse. If you are no longer well enough to have this treatment when it has been made, your doctor might delay your treatment or discuss other treatment options with you.

24.4.3 Step 3: Chemotherapy

If you are still well enough and your CAR T cells have been made successfully, you have chemotherapy to reduce the number of white blood cells in your body. This is to make room for the CAR T cells to multiply in your body. The chemotherapy is given over a few days.

24.4.4 Step 4: CAR T-cell infusion

You usually have only one treatment with CAR T cells. Some people in clinical trials had a second treatment with CAR T cells, but most people had a single treatment. A single treatment should contain enough cells to treat your lymphoma.

The CAR T cells are given intravenously (into a vein).

You are monitored carefully in hospital during and after the treatment. You need to stay close to the hospital you were treated in for at least a month after treatment in case you develop side effects.

24.5 Possible side effects

All medicines can cause side effects (unwanted effects of treatment). As CAR T cells are a new type of treatment, more information about possible side effects is still being gathered.

This is not a complete list of side effects that have been reported. Ask your medical team for the most up-to-date information about possible side effects. Ask all the questions you have. You also need to tell your medical team about any other conditions you have and any medicines, supplements or complementary therapies you are taking before you start any new treatment.

CAR T-cell treatments can cause serious side effects and the treatment is only given in hospitals with the facilities and staff to treat these side effects effectively. You are given treatments to help manage serious side effects before you have the CAR T-cell infusion. These may include paracetamol and antihistamines.

You are monitored closely at the treatment centre as an in-patient for at least a week after having CAR T-cell treatment, and you should look out for new symptoms for at least 4 weeks after having CAR T-cell treatment. You have to stay close to the treatment centre during this time. You should contact your medical team promptly if you have any changes to your health – they will give you more details about what to look out for and who to contact.

Common side effects of CAR T cells, which can affect more than 1 in 5 people, include:
- cytokine release syndrome
- fever and chills

- low blood pressure and low oxygen levels
- nervous system problems, which might include brain problems (encephalopathy), headache, twitching or shaking (tremor), and dizziness
- rapid heart rate (tachycardia) and changes in heart rhythm (arrhythmia)
- fatigue (extreme tiredness)
- cough
- digestive symptoms such as nausea, vomiting, reduced appetite, diarrhoea and constipation
- febrile neutropenia (fever associated with a drop in the number of neutrophils you have – a type of white blood cell that fights infection) and infections.

The most serious of these side effects are described in more detail below.

24.5.1 Cytokine release syndrome

One of the most common and serious complications of CAR T-cell treatments is 'cytokine release syndrome' (CRS). This can happen when CAR T-cell treatment causes a massive immune reaction in your body. This reaction causes the white blood cells affected by the treatment to release substances called 'cytokines' into your blood. Cytokines are proteins that help cells communicate with each other. When they are released, they can signal to other cells to come and help with an immune response. When lots of cytokines are released at once, too many immune cells might be activated at the same time, overwhelming your body.

Symptoms of CRS include fever, chills, low oxygen levels in your body, rapid heart rate and low blood pressure. You are most likely to develop symptoms a couple of days after the CAR T-cell infusion, but they have been known to develop up to 12 days after the infusion.

Almost everyone treated with CAR T-cell treatments experiences some level of CRS due to the way this treatment works. Most cases are mild, and easily treated. Severe, life-threatening reactions can occur. If you have a severe reaction, you might need to be admitted to intensive care for treatments to help with your symptoms, such as oxygen and fluids. You might also be given a drug called 'tocilizumab', which can dampen down the immune response.

24.5.2 Other immune system side effects

As CAR T-cell treatment affects your immune system, you might be at greater risk of infection, including serious infections, after having this treatment. Your white blood cell counts might be low and some people have very low B-cell levels, and low antibody levels (antibodies are proteins that B cells produce to help you fight infection). These problems can make it difficult for your body to fight infections. You might be given drugs such as antibiotics to prevent or treat infections. If you have very low antibody levels, you might need immunoglobulin replacement therapy (infusions of antibodies).

Your medical team can advise you whether your previous vaccinations are still effective, and whether they recommend any vaccinations for you depending on your individual circumstances.

24.5.3 Nervous system problems

Most people treated with CAR T-cell treatments experience nervous system problems within a few days of treatment, although problems can develop up to 8 weeks after treatment. Nervous system problems are usually mild and get better over a couple of weeks. Most commonly, problems develop with the way your brain works, and you may experience headaches, shaking, dizziness, confusion, difficulty sleeping or problems with your speech. Life-threatening problems such as swelling of your brain can develop. Treatments such as steroids can be given if you develop troublesome nervous system problems.

Your medical team will be aware of the signs and symptoms of these side effects and will monitor you closely.

24.6 Precautions

If you have certain other conditions, you might not be able to have CAR T-cell treatment or you might be monitored more carefully. You need to be fit to have this type of treatment.

CAR T-cell treatment has not been approved for use in people under 18 with lymphoma.

People who are pregnant should not usually have CAR T cells during their pregnancy in case it could harm the unborn baby. Your doctor might also advise that you do not breastfeed until you have recovered from the treatment.

Discuss your treatment options with your doctor if you think you might be pregnant.

25 Checkpoint inhibitors

inhibitors, a type of targeted drug used in the treatment of certain types of lymphoma.

25.1 What are checkpoint inhibitors?

Checkpoint inhibitors are a type of targeted treatment that use your own immune system to try to destroy lymphoma cells.

Lymphocytes are white blood cells that are part of your immune system. Your body produces lymphocytes to help you fight infection and disease, including cancer. There are different types of lymphocytes, including T lymphocytes (T cells) and B lymphocytes (B cells), and these have different roles in your immune system. In cancer, cells that become abnormal are not detected by your immune system and can grow out of control. Any type of cell can become cancerous. In lymphoma, cancer develops when lymphocytes themselves become abnormal and are not detected and eliminated by your immune system.

Your T cells usually detect abnormal cells, including cancer cells, and get rid of them. All T cells have proteins called 'T-cell receptors' on their surface, which bind (attach) to other proteins (sometimes called 'antigens') on other cells. When your T-cell receptors bind to another cell, they can 'turn on' your immune system, making it destroy the cells.

T cells also have a different kind of protein that acts as an 'off switch'. These proteins are very important in helping your T cells identify normal, healthy cells, so they do not destroy them. One of these 'off switches' is a protein called 'programmed death-1' (PD-1). PD-1 binds (sticks) to a protein called 'programmed death-1 ligand' (PD-L1) on normal cells, and this interaction (the 'checkpoint') tells the T cell not to destroy the normal cell.

If your own cells become abnormal, they are usually recognised as different by T cells and destroyed by your immune system. Some cancer cells produce PD-L1, which makes them look like normal, healthy cells. The interaction between PD-L1 on the cancer cell and PD-1 on the T cell helps cancer cells avoid being killed by your immune system.

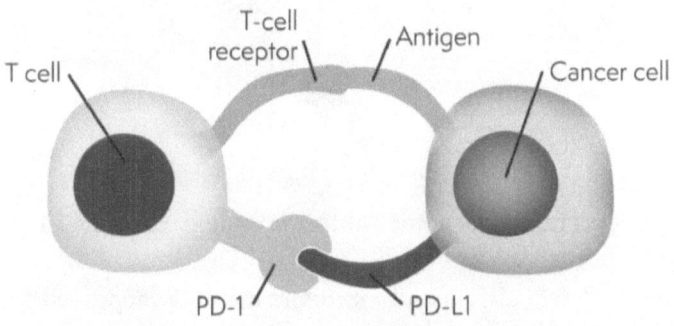

Figure: The PD-1/PD-L1 immune checkpoint with a cancerous, tumour cell

Checkpoint inhibitors work by blocking the PD-1/PD-L1 'checkpoint' and therefore blocking the 'off-switch' for the T cell. This allows the T cells to recognise the lymphoma cells as abnormal, and your immune system can then destroy the lymphoma cells.

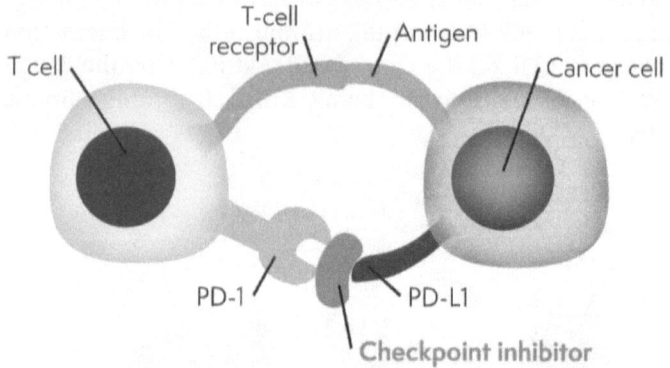

Figure: The checkpoint inhibitor blocks the PD-1/PD-L1 immune checkpoint

There are two checkpoint inhibitors currently approved for use for people with lymphoma in Europe:

- nivolumab (Opdivo®)
- pembrolizumab (Keytruda®).

Both of these drugs bind to PD-1 and block the checkpoint, allowing cancer cells that have PD-L1 to be destroyed by your immune system.

Drugs that block other checkpoints are also in development.

25.2 Who can have them?

Both nivolumab and pembrolizumab are approved in Europe to treat some people with classical Hodgkin lymphoma who have already had other treatments. They are also used to treat some other cancers.

- Nivolumab and pembrolizumab are each recommended for people with classical Hodgkin lymphoma that has relapsed or progressed (got worse) after an autologous stem cell transplant and a different type of targeted treatment, brentuximab vedotin.

- Pembrolizumab can also be used for people with classical Hodgkin lymphoma who cannot have an autologous stem cell transplant and who have already had brentuximab vedotin.

Checkpoint inhibitors are being tested in further clinical trials in people with this type of lymphoma, for example to be used earlier in the treatment pathway. Other checkpoint inhibitors are also being developed and tested. Use our searchable database to see if there is a clinical trial that might be suitable for you at Lymphoma TrialsLink.

25.2.1 Are they available on the NHS in the UK?

Nivolumab and pembrolizumab have been assessed by health authorities for some uses on the NHS in the UK. They are currently only available on the NHS for some people in certain parts of the UK.

In Scotland

- Nivolumab is available on the NHS for people with relapsed or refractory classical Hodgkin lymphoma who have had an autologous stem cell transplant and brentuximab vedotin.
- Pembrolizumab is available on the NHS for people with relapsed or refractory classical Hodgkin lymphoma who have had brentuximab vedotin and a stem cell transplant. It can also be used for people who have had brentuximab vedotin but can't have a stem cell transplant. Pembrolizumab can only be given for up to 2 years.

In England and Wales

- Nivolumab is available on the NHS for people with relapsed or refractory classical Hodgkin lymphoma who have had an autologous stem cell transplant and brentuximab vedotin.

Northern Ireland usually follows NICE recommendations.

In England, pembrolizumab is available through the Cancer Drugs Fund for people with relapsed or refractory classical Hodgkin lymphoma who have had brentuximab vedotin and can't have a stem cell transplant. Pembrolizumab can only be given for up to 2 years.

25.3 Benefits

Results from the main trials that led to approval of nivolumab and pembrolizumab are briefly described below.

25.3.1 Benefits of nivolumab

In several clinical trials, around two-thirds of people with relapsed or refractory classical Hodgkin lymphoma responded to nivolumab (their lymphoma shrank or disappeared completely).

25.3.2 Benefits of pembrolizumab

In a clinical trial of 210 people with relapsed or refractory classical Hodgkin lymphoma, around two-thirds of people responded to pembrolizumab.

25.4 How are they given?

You have nivolumab as an intravenous infusion (into a vein) over 60 minutes. You usually have the treatment once every 2 weeks, where each 2-week period is a 'cycle' of treatment. Most people can have the treatment in hospital as an outpatient, but some people might need to stay overnight for monitoring. It takes an average of 2 months before the benefits of nivolumab are seen. You continue to have nivolumab long-term to keep your lymphoma under control. You can stop treatment if your lymphoma stops responding or you develop side effects that are bad enough to make you stop it.

Pembrolizumab is given in a similar way to nivolumab but the infusion takes 30 minutes and it is usually given once every 3 weeks. You can usually continue to have treatment for up to 2 years if you are being treated on the NHS. You can stop treatment earlier if your lymphoma stops responding or your side effects are not manageable.

25.5 Possible side effects

All medicines can cause side effects (unwanted effects of treatment). As nivolumab and pembrolizumab are new treatments, more information about possible side effects is still being gathered.

The most common side effects of both drugs, which can affect more than 1 in 10 people, are:

- digestive problems, such as diarrhoea and nausea
- rash and itching
- fatigue (extreme tiredness).

These side effects are not usually severe.

Immune-related side effects can occur, due to the immune system causing inflammation of your organs. These can include problems with your lungs, bowel, liver, kidneys and thyroid. These side effects can usually be treated with steroids or go away when you stop treatment with checkpoint inhibitors. In some cases, problems can be severe and some people take a long time to recover.

Severe infusion-related reactions (occur while the treatment is given or shortly afterwards) can develop that make people feel very ill and require prompt treatment. Symptoms of infusion reactions include fever, chills, shaking, dizziness and itching. If you have an infusion reaction, you are monitored carefully and the checkpoint inhibitor treatment might be stopped.

This is not a complete list of side effects that have been reported. Ask your medical team for the most up-to-date information about possible side effects. Ask all the questions you have. You also need to tell your medical team about any other conditions you have and any medicines, supplements or complementary therapies you are taking before you start any new treatment.

Your medical team monitor you closely for side effects during treatment. They can tell you what to look out for and who to contact if you have any problems.

25.6 Precautions

You might not be able to have checkpoint inhibitors if you are taking other medications or have other conditions.

Make sure you tell your doctor about any medical conditions and any medicines you are taking.

Your doctor may reduce your dose and monitor you more closely or recommend that you do not have checkpoint inhibitors if you have problems such as autoimmune conditions (where your body attacks itself) or serious lung problems. Your doctor might also change your dose if you experience troublesome side effects.

Checkpoint inhibitors have not been approved for use in people under 18.

If you are pregnant, you should not usually have checkpoint inhibitors during pregnancy in case they could harm your unborn baby. You must use effective measures of contraception to prevent pregnancy during treatment and you should not breastfeed. Discuss your treatment options with your doctor if you think you might be pregnant.

26 Ibrutinib

ibrutinib in the treatment of lymphoma.

26.1 What is ibrutinib?

Many newer treatments for lymphoma are targeted drugs.

Targeted drugs aim to kill the type of cell that has turned cancerous or stop signals that make cancerous cells grow or divide. In lymphoma, the type of cell that becomes cancerous is called a 'lymphocyte' (a type of white blood cell that fights infection). There are several types of lymphocyte that can become cancerous. Ibrutinib targets B lymphocytes (B cells) and is therefore used to treat B-cell lymphomas.

Cells send and receive signals to other cells. Some of these signals keep cells alive and make them divide. There are lots of signalling pathways and signals are sent along one or more of these pathways. Ibrutinib (Imbruvica®) is a cell signal blocker<LINK> that targets a protein called 'Bruton's tyrosine kinase' (BTK). BTK is a part of a pathway that helps B cells to stay alive and divide. Blocking BTK can make B cells die or prevent them dividing. This treatment can therefore stop the spread of cancerous B cells.

26.2 Who can have ibrutinib?

Ibrutinib is approved in Europe for treating three types of lymphoma.

Mantle cell lymphoma

- For people whose lymphoma has relapsed (come back) or has not responded to treatment (refractory lymphoma). Ibrutinib is given on its own.

Chronic lymphocytic leukaemia (CLL)

- For people who have not yet had treatment for their CLL (first-line treatment). Ibrutinib is given on its own.
- For people whose CLL has relapsed after treatment. For people with relapsed CLL, ibrutinib can be given on its own or with bendamustine (a chemotherapy drug) and rituximab (an antibody treatment).

Waldenström's macroglobulinaemia (WM)

- For people who have previously received other treatments for WM. Ibrutinib is given on its own.
- For people who can't have chemo-immunotherapy (chemotherapy with antibody therapy) as first-line treatment. Ibrutinib is given on its own.

European approval to use ibrutinib in CLL and mantle cell lymphoma was granted in November 2014. It was then extended to WM in May 2015. In 2016, the European Medicines Agency (EMA) expanded ibrutinib's recommended uses for CLL.

Ibrutinib is being tested in further clinical trials in people with these types of lymphoma. This is to see if ibrutinib could work better in combination with other treatments, such as chemotherapy or antibody therapy (for example, rituximab). It is also being tested in other types of lymphoma. Use our searchable database to see if there's a clinical trial that might be suitable for you at Lymphoma TrialsLink.

26.2.1 Is it available on the NHS in the UK?

Ibrutinib has been assessed by health authorities for some uses on the NHS in the UK. It is currently only available on the NHS for some people in certain parts of the UK.

In Scotland

- For people with relapsed or refractory mantle cell lymphoma.
- For people with relapsed or refractory CLL who can't have treatments that include fludarabine.
- For people with CLL and a 17p deletion (a genetic change that means the CLL does not respond well to chemo-immunotherapy).

In England and Wales

- For people with relapsed or refractory mantle cell lymphoma who have only had one previous course of treatment.
- For people with CLL who have had previous treatment or who have a 17p deletion or TP53 mutation (genetic changes that mean the CLL does not respond well to chemo-immunotherapy).

- Through the Cancer Drugs Fund for people with relapsed or refractory WM.

Ibrutinib is also being assessed by the National Institute for Health and Care Excellence (NICE) for other uses, for example in combination with different treatments for certain types of lymphoma.

Northern Ireland usually follows NICE recommendations.

26.3 Benefits

Ibrutinib is considered by many experts to be a 'breakthrough treatment' for some types of lymphoma. It gives higher response rates compared with other therapies for the same types of lymphoma. The main trials that led to approval of ibrutinib are briefly described below.

26.3.1 Benefits in mantle cell lymphoma

Mantle cell lymphoma that has relapsed or not responded to first-line therapy can be difficult to treat. However, the main study in this area showed that more than two-thirds of 111 people treated with ibrutinib responded to the treatment (their lymphoma shrank or disappeared).

A second study in 280 people compared ibrutinib with another cancer drug, temsirolimus, in people with relapsed or refractory mantle cell lymphoma. People lived for an average of 15 months without their lymphoma getting worse when treated with ibrutinib compared with an average of 6 months when treated with temsirolimus.

26.3.2 Benefits in chronic lymphocytic leukaemia (CLL)

Long-lasting responses have been seen in people with CLL treated with ibrutinib. In the main trial involving 391 people with relapsed or refractory CLL, ibrutinib was compared with ofatumumab, which is often used for people with CLL that has come back. One year after starting treatment, around 66 in 100 people taking ibrutinib had CLL that had stayed under control (this is called 'progression-free survival') compared with around 6 in 100 people treated with ofatumumab.

In a second study involving 269 people who hadn't yet received any treatment for their CLL, ibrutinib was compared with the chemotherapy drug chlorambucil. After 1.5 years of treatment, around 90 in 100 people taking ibrutinib had CLL that had stayed under control compared with around 52 in 100 people treated with chlorambucil.

Adding ibrutinib to bendamustine and rituximab for people with relapsed or refractory CLL was also effective in a study involving 578 people. The risk of CLL progressing was reduced by taking ibrutinib instead of a placebo (dummy treatment).

26.3.3 Benefits in Waldenström's macroglobulinaemia (WM)

A high response rate has also been seen in people with WM – about 9 in 10 people with WM responded to ibrutinib treatment in a trial in 63 people. This trial was a significant breakthrough for WM as it is an uncommon form of lymphoma and it is therefore difficult to recruit enough people to take part in a clinical trial. This trial led to the approval of ibrutinib for WM in Europe.

26.4 How is it given?

Ibrutinib is given as capsules which are taken orally (by mouth). Always follow the advice of your medical team when taking ibrutinib. You can usually take the capsules at home. Make sure you know how many capsules you should take – your recommended dose of ibrutinib is based on the type of lymphoma you have and your general health.

- Swallow the capsules whole with a glass of water.
- Never open the capsules, break them or chew them.
- Take the capsules at about the same time every day.
- Check the information you are given to find out what you should do if you miss a dose.

26.4.1 When is ibrutinib given?

Ibrutinib capsules are taken once daily. They can be taken every day until your lymphoma stops responding unless side effects are bad enough to make you stop treatment. You might be treated with ibrutinib for years.

Keep taking ibrutinib for as long as your medical team tells you to, even if you feel well. If ibrutinib is keeping your lymphoma under control, the lymphoma could get worse if you stop taking the drug.

26.4.2 Will I need any special tests while I am taking ibrutinib?

You will need to have blood tests to check your health, for example your blood cell counts, while you are taking ibrutinib. Your medical team might want you to have other tests depending on any other conditions you have or any side effects you develop. For example, you might have an electrocardiogram (ECG; a heart function test that records the rhythm and electrical activity of the heart) to check how well your heart is working. How often you need these tests depends on your individual circumstances such as other health conditions you have and how your lymphoma is responding.

26.5 Possible side effects

All medicines can cause side effects (unwanted effects of treatment).

Only the most common side effects of ibrutinib are described on this page. This is not a complete list of side effects that have been reported. As ibrutinib is a new treatment, more information about possible side effects is still being gathered. There is limited information about late effects (side effects that only develop months or years after treatment has finished) of ibrutinib. Your team should discuss the most up-to-date information with you before you start treatment. Ask all the questions you have. Discuss with your medical team how ibrutinib might affect any other medical conditions you have. You also need to tell your medical team about any medicines, supplements or complementary therapies you are taking before you start any new treatment.

Most side effects experienced by people treated with ibrutinib are mild. In clinical studies, few people (about 5 in 100) had to reduce their dose of ibrutinib because of side effects. A similar number (about 5 in 100) had to stop treatment for this reason. Some side effects, such as diarrhoea, tend to occur early in treatment and then settle down if you continue to take ibrutinib, without **needing** to reduce your dose.

The most common side effects of ibrutinib, which can affect more than 1 in 5 people, are:

- neutropenia (low neutrophils), which increases your risk of infection
- gastrointestinal effects: nausea, diarrhoea
- musculoskeletal pain (pain in muscles and bones)
- bruising and bleeding
- rash
- fever.

Some of these risks are described in more detail below.

Although minor bleeding problems (for example bruising) are common, more serious events (for example a haemorrhage) can occur less commonly. Changes in heart rhythm can also present. These effects are described below.

26.5.1 Effects on blood

Ibrutinib can decrease the number of different types of cells in your blood. These effects are usually mild but can result in an increased risk of bleeding and developing infections. Ibrutinib can also cause a temporary increase in the number of lymphocytes (a type of white blood cell) in your blood. This does not normally cause any problems. Your medical team will check your blood cell counts regularly.

26.5.2 Bleeding problems

Ibrutinib can cause bleeding problems. These can be minor, such as bruising more easily, or serious, such as a haemorrhage. Bleeding problems could be caused by the effects of ibrutinib on platelet function. Platelets are found in your blood and help it to clot. It is not known why some people develop bleeding problems while others do not.

People who take other drugs that affect platelets or drugs that thin the blood (anticoagulants such as warfarin) might not be able to take ibrutinib or may be monitored more carefully.

Tell your medical team if you notice any symptoms of bleeding problems so that you can receive prompt treatment: bloody or black stools (they look like tar), pink or brown urine, unexpected bleeding or bleeding that is severe or that you cannot control, vomiting blood or vomit that looks like coffee grounds, coughing up blood or blood clots, increased bruising, feeling dizzy or weak, confusion, changes in your speech, or a long-lasting headache. Your medical team might need to adjust your dose of ibrutinib or stop treatment if you experience significant bleeding problems.

26.5.3 Infections

Treatment with ibrutinib can lower your number of neutrophils (a type of white blood cell that fights infection). If you have neutropenia (low neutrophils), you may be at higher risk of getting an infection. Neutropenia experienced with ibrutinib is generally mild. People treated with ibrutinib commonly get infections including colds, sore throats and sinus infections. More serious infections, for example pneumonia, can occur.

It is also possible for infections that usually remain dormant in your body to flare up during treatment with ibrutinib. You might need extra monitoring if you have ever had hepatitis B (a liver infection).

26.5.4 Heart problems

Some people treated with ibrutinib develop heart rhythm problems. These are more likely in people who are at a higher risk of heart problems or who have had them in the past. In many cases, changes in heart rhythm are mild so you can continue taking ibrutinib but you may need to be monitored more carefully. Tell your medical team immediately if:

- you feel like your heart is beating quickly and irregularly
- you are light-headed, dizzy or faint
- you have shortness of breath or any discomfort in your chest.

Your medical team will consider carefully whether ibrutinib is suitable for you if you already have heart rhythm problems or a relevant family history.

26.6 Who can't have ibrutinib?

Some people will not be able to have ibrutinib because they are taking other medications or have other conditions. Make sure you tell your medical team about any medical conditions and any medicines you are taking. Your medical team may reduce your dose and monitor you more closely or recommend that you do not take ibrutinib if you have other conditions. These include liver problems, severe kidney problems or severe heart disease.

Some medications, including herbal remedies, can interact with ibrutinib and should not be taken with it. They could increase the risk of side effects or change the effect of ibrutinib. Give your medical team a list of all the medications you are taking. Make sure you include any vitamins, supplements or herbal remedies.

Drugs that affect blood clotting: At the moment, it is not recommended that ibrutinib is given with warfarin. Ibrutinib can be given with some other medicines that thin your blood or stop it from clotting but you will need to be monitored carefully because of an increased risk of bleeding. If you are taking warfarin, your medical team is likely to recommend that you change to a different blood-thinning medicine if you need to take ibrutinib. You shouldn't take certain vitamins and supplements, such as fish oil or vitamin E.

Drugs that affect an enzyme called CYP3A4: CYP3A4 acts on many drugs to help remove them from the body, including ibrutinib. If you are taking a drug that interferes with the action of CYP3A4, it can decrease or increase the action of ibrutinib, depending on how the drugs work together. It is important that your medical team knows about all the medications you are taking as there is a range of drugs that can have this effect, including some antibiotics and herbal remedies such as St John's Wort (used for depression and anxiety).

If you are about to have or have recently had surgery, you will not be able to take ibrutinib for at least 3 to 7 days before and after your operation, depending on the type of surgery recommended and your risk of bleeding.

Ibrutinib has not been approved for use in people under 18. You must not take ibrutinib if you are pregnant or become pregnant as it could damage your unborn baby. Discuss your treatment options with your medical team if you think you might be pregnant.

26.7 Precautions

You might need to take certain precautions while being treated with ibrutinib.

Certain drugs and foods can increase your risk of side effects during treatment with ibrutinib.

- Tell your medical team if you are taking or would like to start taking any medications including, but not limited to, vitamins, supplements and herbal remedies.
- Don't drink grapefruit juice or eat grapefruit or Seville oranges (including if it is used in marmalade). These can increase the amounts of ibrutinib in your blood.

Report any side effects to your medical team as soon as possible. Your team might be able to give you medicine or advice to help with troublesome side effects.

- Follow your medical team's advice if you have low blood counts.
- Do not drive or operate any machinery if you have side effects such as fatigue or dizziness.
- Drink plenty of fluids. Diarrhoea is common in people taking ibrutinib but usually goes away after a couple of days. Tell your medical team if your diarrhoea does not go away in a couple of weeks.

Ibrutinib could damage an unborn baby or be passed to your baby in breast milk. Below are some recommendations you should follow.

- Prevent getting pregnant during treatment and for at least 3 months afterwards.

- Use a barrier method of contraception, such as condoms. The effect of ibrutinib on hormonal contraceptives, for example the pill, is unknown.
- Do not breastfeed if you are taking ibrutinib.

27 Idelalisib

idelalisib, a targeted drug used in the treatment of certain types of lymphoma.

27.1 What is idelalisib?

Many newer treatments for lymphoma are targeted drugs.

Targeted drugs aim to kill the type of cell that has turned cancerous or stop signals that make cancerous cells grow or divide. In lymphoma, the type of cell that becomes cancerous is called a 'lymphocyte' (a type of white blood cell that fights infection). There are several types of lymphocyte, such as B lymphocytes (B cells) and T lymphocytes (T cells), which can be targeted by these newer treatments.

Cells receive signals that keep them alive and make them divide. These signals are sent along one or more signalling pathways inside the body. Idelalisib (Zydelig®) is a cell signal blocker. It targets a protein called 'phosphatidylinositol 3-kinase' (PI3K), which is one of the steps in a pathway that helps B cells to stay alive and divide. This pathway is particularly important in helping cancerous B cells (lymphoma cells) stay alive when they should have died. Blocking the PI3K pathway with idelalisib can stop lymphoma cells dividing or cause them to die, stopping the spread of the lymphoma.

Idelalisib was previously known as GS-1101 or CAL-101.

27.2 Who can have it?

At the time of writing, idelalisib is approved in Europe for the following types of lymphoma.

Chronic lymphocytic leukaemia (CLL)/small lymphocytic lymphoma (SLL)

- For people who have had previous treatment for CLL/SLL. Idelalisib is given with rituximab or ofatumumab (both antibody treatments).
- For people with genetic changes in their cells that make their CLL/SLL harder to treat (called '17p deletion', where some genes are missing) and who are unable to have other treatments, such as chemotherapy. Idelalisib is given with rituximab or ofatumumab.
- Follicular lymphoma
- For people whose follicular lymphoma is refractory (not responding to treatment) after at least two previous treatments. Idelalisib is given on its own.

Idelalisib is also being tested in clinical trials for various types of lymphoma. Visit our clinical trials information service, Lymphoma TrialsLink to find out more about clinical trials and to search our database for a clinical trial that might be suitable for you.

27.2.1 Is it available on the NHS in the UK?

Idelalisib has been assessed by health authorities for some uses on the NHS in the UK. It is currently only available on the NHS for some people in certain parts of the UK.

In Scotland

- Idelalisib can be used in combination with rituximab for people who have had previous treatment for CLL/SLL and who are not able to have chemotherapy.
- Idelalisib can be used as a first-line treatment in combination with rituximab for people with genetic changes in their cells that make their CLL/SLL harder to treat (17p deletion, where some genes are missing).
- Idelalisib can be used for people who have had at least two previous courses of treatment for follicular lymphoma.

In England and Wales

- Idelalisib can be used in combination with rituximab for people who have had previous treatment for CLL/SLL but whose CLL/SLL has got worse within 2 years of their previous treatment.
- Idelalisib can be used for people with CLL/SLL who have genetic changes in their cells that make their condition harder to treat (17p deletion, where some genes are missing) and who are unable to have other treatments.
- Idelalisib is currently being assessed for use on the NHS for people with follicular lymphoma, and a decision is expected in February 2019.

Northern Ireland usually follows National Institute for Health and Care Excellence (NICE) recommendations, which cover England and Wales.

27.3 Benefits

27.3.1 Benefits in CLL/SLL

Idelalisib was shown to be very effective at treating CLL/SLL in a clinical trial of 220 people who had previously received treatment. This trial compared idelalisib in combination with rituximab with placebo (a dummy treatment instead of idelalisib) in combination with rituximab. Three in four people treated with idelalisib and rituximab responded to treatment (their CLL/SLL improved). Only around one in every seven people treated with placebo (a dummy treatment) and rituximab responded to treatment. Some of the people in this trial had genetic changes that make their CLL more difficult to treat, and these people also responded better to idelalisib and rituximab than to placebo and rituximab.

Idelalisib is also effective in treating CLL in combination with another antibody treatment, called ofatumumab. In a study of 261 people who had received previous treatment for their CLL, the disease stayed under control for twice as long in people who had idelalisib with ofatumumab compared with those who had ofatumumab alone.

27.3.2 Benefits in follicular lymphoma

Around half of people who had at least two previous courses of treatment for follicular lymphoma responded to idelalisib in a trial that included 72 people with follicular lymphoma.

27.4 How is it given?

Idelalisib is taken as tablets. Always follow the advice of your doctor when taking idelalisib. You can usually take the treatment at home.

You take idelalisib twice a day.

You take idelalisib every day until your lymphoma stops responding to it, unless side effects are bad enough to make you stop treatment. You might be treated with idelalisib for years.

Keep taking idelalisib for as long as your doctor tells you to, even if you feel well. If idelalisib is keeping your lymphoma under control, the lymphoma could get worse if you stop taking the drug.

27.5 Possible side effects

All medicines can cause side effects (unwanted effects of treatment).

Only the most common side effects of idelalisib are described on this page. This is not a complete list of side effects that have been reported. As idelalisib is a new treatment, more information about possible side effects is still being gathered. There is limited information about late effects (side effects that only develop months or years after treatment has finished) of idelalisib. Your medical team should discuss the most up-to-date information about side effects with you before you start treatment. Ask all the questions you have.

Tell your medical team about any other medical conditions you have, as you might need additional monitoring or changes to the management of other conditions if you are treated with idelalisib. You must also tell your medical team about any medicines, supplements or complementary therapies you are taking before you start any new treatment.

Most side effects experienced by people treated with idelalisib are mild. Tell your medical team if you notice any changes in your health. You might need to take a lower dose of idelalisib or stop treatment temporarily if you are having troublesome side effects, or you might need other treatments to help with side effects.

Most common side effects (occur in more than 1 in 10 people):
- increased risk of infections, including serious infections like pneumonia, cytomegalovirus and fungal infections
- neutropenia (low neutrophils, a type of white blood cell that fights infection)
- lymphocytosis (increased levels of lymphocytes – this does not normally cause any problems)
- diarrhoea
- rash
- fever
- increased blood fat levels, and increased liver enzymes in blood tests (which can indicate problems with your liver).

Less common but possibly serious side effects:
- pneumonitis (inflammation of the lungs)
- colitis (inflammation of the large intestine)
- Stevens-Johnson syndrome or Toxic Epidermal Necrolysis (serious skin disorders).

Some people treated with idelalisib have developed colitis months after treatment started. Tell your doctor if you experience any new or worsening diarrhoea. If you develop colitis, your idelalisib treatment might be stopped temporarily and treatments given to help your symptoms, such as anti-inflammatory drugs.

Several clinical trials with idelalisib were stopped because of people getting serious infections. This was more likely to happen when idelalisib was used together with other drugs. However, the European Medicines Agency's (EMA) Committee for Medicinal Products for Human Use (CHMP) concluded after review that the benefits of idelalisib outweighed the risk of side effects in CLL and follicular lymphoma. Measures have been put in place to reduce the risk of infection. If you are taking idelalisib, your doctor monitors you for infection. You will also given antibiotics during and after treatment to prevent a serious infection developing.

27.6 Precautions

You might need to take certain precautions while being treated with idelalisib.

Lots of medications, including herbal remedies, can interact with idelalisib and should not be taken with it. They could increase the risk of side effects or change the effect of idelalisib. Give your doctor a list of all the medications you are taking. Make sure you include any vitamins, supplements or herbal remedies. Tell your doctor if you are considering starting any new medications before you start.

Drugs that affect an enzyme called CYP3A4: CYP3A4 acts on many drugs to help remove them from the body, including idelalisib. If you are taking a drug that interferes with the action of CYP3A4, it can decrease or increase the action of idelalisib, depending on how the drugs work together. It is important that your doctor knows about all the medications you are taking as there is a range of drugs that can affect idelalisib.

Report any side effects to your doctor as soon as possible. Your doctor might be able to give you medicine or advice to help with troublesome side effects.

Idelalisib has not been approved for use in people under 18.

Idelalisib could damage an unborn baby or be passed to your baby in breast milk. Below are some recommendations you should follow.

- Prevent getting pregnant during treatment and for at least 1 month afterwards.
- Use a barrier method of contraception, like condoms. The effect of idelalisib on hormonal contraceptives, for example the pill, is unknown.
- Do not breastfeed if you are taking idelalisib.

28 Venetoclax

venetoclax, a targeted drug used in the treatment of certain types of low-grade (slow-growing) lymphoma.

28.1 What is venetoclax?

Venetoclax (Venclyxto®) is a targeted drug that can make lymphoma cells undergo apoptosis (programmed cell death).

When cells are no longer needed, for example when they're damaged, they die in a controlled way. This is called 'apoptosis' and it is a normal process within the body. Cancer can occur when there is a build-up of cells that survived when they should have died.

Venetoclax switches off the survival signals that keep some types of cancer cells alive when they should have died. This can make the cancer cells die.

28.2 Who can have it?

Venetoclax is approved in Europe for some people with chronic lymphocytic leukaemia (CLL):

- People with CLL that has certain genetic changes (17p deletion or TP53 mutation) and who can't have a different type of targeted drug, a B-cell receptor pathway inhibitor (ibrutinib or idelalisib), or their condition didn't respond to these drugs.
- People with CLL that didn't respond to both chemo-immunotherapy (chemotherapy with antibody therapy) and a B-cell receptor pathway inhibitor (ibrutinib or idelalisib).

In combination with rituximab, venetoclax is also licensed for people with CLL who didn't respond to at least one previous treatment.

Venetoclax is being tested in further clinical trials in people with CLL to see if combining it with other treatments makes it more effective. It is also being tested in other types of lymphoma. Use our searchable database to see if there's a clinical trial that might be suitable for you at Lymphoma TrialsLink.

28.2.1 Is it available on the NHS in the UK?

Venetoclax has been assessed by health authorities for use on the NHS in the UK and is currently available on its own throughout the UK. In combination with rituximab, venetoclax is available in England, Wales and Northern Ireland. The combination is currently being assessed in Scotland.

Venetoclax is also being assessed for other uses, for example in combination with different treatments for certain types of lymphoma.

28.3 Benefits

Venetoclax is becoming increasingly important as a treatment for CLL. It is currently used if other targeted drugs have failed to keep CLL under control.

Venetoclax gives high response rates and can completely clear CLL in some people – this is called a 'complete remission'. A complete remission makes it more likely that your CLL will stay under control for a long time.

In the main clinical trial of 107 people with relapsed CLL and 17p deletion, three-quarters of people responded to treatment (their CLL was reduced or completely disappeared). In a clinical trial of 64 people with CLL who had previously taken idelalisib or ibrutinib, around two-thirds responded to treatment.

28.4 How is it given?

You take venetoclax as tablets once a day with a meal. You start at a low dose and the dose is gradually increased over the first 5 weeks of treatment. This reduces the number of CLL cells gradually. Killing too many cells at once can cause a serious side effect called 'tumour lysis syndrome', as your kidneys can struggle to remove the high levels of waste products from dying cells. Your dose may be reduced if you have troublesome side effects.

You keep taking venetoclax for as long as it is benefitting you and until your CLL stops responding to it. You may stop taking venetoclax earlier than this if you develop problematic side effects. This means you might continue to take venetoclax for several years, although some studies are testing whether venetoclax can be stopped after you have been in remission for a certain amount of time, without your CLL coming back.

28.5 Possible side effects

All medicines can cause side effects (unwanted effects of treatment). As venetoclax is a new treatment, more information about possible side effects is still being gathered.

This is not a complete list of side effects that have been reported. Ask your medical team for the most up-to-date information about possible side effects. Ask all the questions you have. You also need to tell your medical team about any other conditions you have and any medicines, supplements or complementary therapies you are taking before you start any new treatment.

The most common side effects of venetoclax, which can affect more than 1 in 5 people, are:

- neutropenia (a drop in the number of neutrophils you have – a type of white blood cell that fights infection)
- gastrointestinal problems, such as nausea and vomiting, diarrhoea and constipation
- anaemia (a drop in the number of red blood cells you have)
- infections (for example, colds)
- abnormally high levels of phosphate in your blood, which might mean your kidneys are not working properly
- fatigue (extreme tiredness).

Less common but serious side effects can include:

- neutropenic sepsis (fever associated with neutropenia)
- serious infections like pneumonia.

Tumour lysis syndrome (TLS)

One possible complication of treatment with venetoclax is tumour lysis syndrome, which is problems caused by the rapid breakdown of cancer cells. To reduce the risk of TLS, your dose of venetoclax is increased gradually and you are monitored carefully.

- You should make sure you drink plenty of water before starting venetoclax and while your dose is being increased. Some people are given intravenous fluids (into a vein).
- You may be given other medications to reduce the risk of tumour lysis syndrome, or be monitored in hospital.
- You have regular blood tests so that tumour lysis syndrome can be detected quickly and venetoclax can be stopped. You might be able to restart venetoclax at the same dose or at a reduced dose.

Your medical team can give you further advice about fluid intake and reducing the risk of tumour lysis syndrome.

28.6 Precautions

You might not be able to have venetoclax if you are taking other medications or have certain other conditions. Your doctor may reduce your dose and monitor you more closely or recommend that you do not take venetoclax if you have other conditions. These include liver problems and kidney problems. Your doctor might also change your dose if you experience troublesome side effects.

Certain drugs and foods can increase your risk of side effects during treatment with venetoclax.

- **Drugs that affect an enzyme called CYP3A4**: CYP3A4 acts on many drugs to help remove them from the body, including venetoclax. If you are taking a drug that interferes with the action of CYP3A4, it can decrease or increase the action of venetoclax, depending on how the drugs work together. It is important that your doctor knows about all the medications you are taking as there is a range of drugs that can have this effect, including some antibiotics and herbal remedies such as St John's Wort (used for depression and anxiety).

- **Don't drink grapefruit juice or eat grapefruit or Seville oranges** (used in some types of marmalade). These can increase the amounts of venetoclax in your blood.

Venetoclax has not been approved for use in people under 18.

People who are pregnant should not usually have venetoclax during their pregnancy in case it could harm the unborn baby. Below are some recommendations you should follow.

- Prevent getting pregnant during treatment and for at least 30 days after finishing venetoclax treatment.
- Use a barrier method of contraception, like condoms. The effect of venetoclax on hormonal contraceptives, for example the pill, is unknown.
- Do not breastfeed if you are taking venetoclax.

Discuss your treatment options with your doctor if you think you might be pregnant.

29 Other targeted drugs for lymphoma

29.1 Types of targeted drugs

Some targeted drugs are in routine use for people with lymphoma in the UK. There are others that are approved for use in Europe but not yet funded on the NHS in the UK, or that are not yet used for many people with lymphoma. These drugs can still be used in the UK for certain people, but might need to be funded outside of the NHS. The sections below describe some of the other targeted drugs that are approved for use in Europe and how they work.

Different ways to target lymphoma cells are under investigation. This page is updated regularly to include new drugs approved for people with lymphoma.

29.2 Radioimmunotherapy

Radioimmunotherapy uses an antibody (immunotherapy) to deliver a small dose of radiation (radiotherapy) directly to lymphoma cells. Targeting radiotherapy to the lymphoma cells means it causes less harm to normal cells.

Zevalin® is the only radioimmunotherapy treatment currently approved to treat lymphoma in Europe.

29.2.1 Zevalin® (90Y-ibritumomab tiuxetan)

Zevalin® is ibritumomab (an antibody which targets the protein CD20, which is found on lymphoma cells) joined to a radioactive particle, yttrium-90.

Who can have it?
Zevalin® is approved in Europe for some people with follicular lymphoma.

It is approved to treat:

- People who have gone into remission (no evidence of follicular lymphoma) after their first course of chemo-immunotherapy (chemotherapy with antibody treatment). It aims to give a longer-lasting remission – this is called 'consolidation'.
- People whose follicular lymphoma has relapsed (come back) after treatment containing rituximab or whose lymphoma is no longer responding to treatment containing rituximab(refractory).

However, it is not currently available on the NHS in the UK and has not been assessed by NICE for use in the UK.

How is it given?
Zevalin® is only given at certain hospitals as it requires specially trained staff and specialist facilities. It is given intravenously (into a vein) over 10 minutes. You have a single dose of Zevalin®. A low dose of rituximab is given 7 to 9 days before Zevalin®. A second dose of rituximab is given just before Zevalin®.

29.3 Cell signal blockers
Cells receive signals that keep them alive and make them divide. These signals are sent along different signalling pathways inside the body. Blocking either the signal or a key part of the pathway can make cells die or stop the lymphoma from growing. Certain signalling pathways are more important in some types of lymphoma than in others. Scientists don't yet fully understand how all the various pathways are linked.

Some cell signal blockers are already in routine use for some types of lymphoma, such as ibrutinib and idelalisib.

There is one cell signal blocker approved for use for people with lymphoma but not funded on the NHS: temsirolimus (Torisel®).

There are many other cell signal blockers in development and in clinical trials for people with lymphoma.

29.3.1 Temsirolimus (Torisel®)

Temsirolimus targets a pathway known as 'mammalian target of rapamycin' (mTOR), which helps lymphoma cells to divide. Blocking this pathway can stop lymphoma cells spreading.

Who can have it?
Temsirolimus is approved in Europe for people with mantle cell lymphoma whose lymphoma has relapsed (come back) or is refractory (didn't respond well) to other treatments.

It is not funded on the NHS in the UK.

How is it given?
Temsirolimus is given intravenously (into a vein) over about 30 to 60 minutes once a week. Treatment usually continues until the lymphoma stops responding unless you are not tolerating the treatment (you have severe side effects).

29.4 Proteasome inhibitors

There are lots of different proteins in cells which help to control normal processes, including how cells divide (make new cells). Proteasomes break down proteins in cells and this keeps a balance of proteins in the cell. This is a normal process but also occurs in abnormal cells to keep them alive, for example lymphoma cells. Proteasome inhibitors block the work of proteasomes. This seems to be particularly harmful to certain types of lymphoma cells, which are then no longer able to work properly and die.

The only proteasome inhibitor currently approved to treat people with lymphoma in Europe is bortezomib.

29.4.1 Bortezomib (Bortezomib Accord or Velcade®)

Bortezomib blocks the work of proteasomes.

Who can have it?
Bortezomib is approved in Europe to treat people with mantle cell lymphoma who cannot have a stem cell transplant. It is given with chemo-immunotherapy (rituximab, cyclophosphamide, doxorubicin and prednisone, known as R-CHP) as a first-line treatment for people who have not yet had treatment. It is funded on the NHS in the UK for this use.

How is it given?
Bortezomib is given intravenously (into the vein) or subcutaneously (by injection just under the skin). It is usually given twice a week for 2 weeks followed by a 10 day rest period in each 3-week cycle. A total of 6 to 8 cycles are usually given for people with mantle cell lymphoma that has not been treated previously.

29.5 Immunomodulators

Immunomodulators are believed to work by changing how the immune system works. They can do this in different ways, for example, by:

- restoring some of the signals between immune system cells and lymphoma cells
- blocking some of the signals within lymphoma cells.

The only immunomodulator currently approved to treat people with lymphoma in Europe is lenalidomide.

29.5.1 Lenalidomide (Revlimid®)

Lenalidomide is an immunomodulatory drug. It affects the activity of the immune system in several different ways, both in helping the immune system to attack the lymphoma cells and in preventing the lymphoma from growing.

Who can have it?
Lenalidomide is approved in Europe for people with relapsed or refractory mantle cell lymphoma. It is not currently funded on the NHS.

How is it given?
Lenalidomide is taken as tablets once a day for 21 days, followed by 7 days without treatment in each 28-day cycle. Cycles of treatment are usually repeated until the lymphoma stops responding unless unless you are not tolerating the treatment (you have severe side effects).

30 Side effects of lymphoma treatment

Side effects of treatments for lymphoma

Side effects you may experience during treatment for lymphoma.

30.1 What are side effects of treatment?

The aim of treatment for lymphoma is to destroy all of the lymphoma cells. However, all treatments for lymphoma have other, unwanted effects on the body, which are called 'side effects'.

Treatments for lymphoma affect everyone differently. Each type of treatment or drug has a different set of possible side effects. The dose and treatment schedule (how often you have the drug or treatment) and the combination of treatments you have affect what side effects you get. Side effects also vary in how severe they are; some people have only mild side effects while others have more troublesome effects. Although some side effects for each treatment are common, not everyone gets them.

It is difficult to predict how a treatment may affect you. However, before you start any treatment, it is very important that you tell your doctor about any medical conditions you have other than lymphoma. Some conditions mean you could have more serious side effects with certain treatments.

You must also tell your doctor about any other treatments you are taking, including drugs, vitamins and herbal remedies. Drugs can interact with each other, which might make them more or less effective. These interactions could also cause very serious side effects.

Side effects tend to be short-term, but some can last for a few weeks or months after treatment has finished (long-term side effects), eg fatigue and peripheral neuropathy. Occasionally, side effects may be permanent. Some side effects can occur later in life (late effects).

30.2 What are the most common side effects of lymphoma treatments?

Each treatment has its own set of most common side effects. Ask your doctor for information on the possible side effects of any treatments they recommend. Talk to your medical team if you are having any side effects even if they seem minor. Your medical team want to help make your treatment as comfortable as possible for you. They can offer tailored advice to help you cope with your symptoms. There are often treatments available that can help with side effects or it might be possible to change your treatment slightly, eg reduce the speed at which a drug is given.

Our pages provide practical advice on dealing with specific side effects. This is not a comprehensive list of the side effects you might have. There are many, less common side effects that we do not mention here..

We also have information about diet and nutrition, which includes suggestions to help with eating problems that commonly affect people who are having treatment for lymphoma.

Some symptoms occur in many people treated for lymphoma. These can be side effects of treatment or may be caused by the lymphoma itself, for example:

- fatigue

- cancer-related cognitive impairment ('chemo brain').

30.2.1 Side effects of chemotherapy

There are some side effects that are common for many types of chemotherapy. Because chemotherapy drugs work by killing any dividing cells, they can damage healthy cells as well as lymphoma cells. It is this damage to healthy cells that causes many of the side effects of chemotherapy. Healthy cells in the body that are dividing include those in the gut, the hair follicles and the bone marrow, which is why the following side effects are common:

- nausea and vomiting
- hair loss
- lowered blood counts:
  neutropenia, anaemia and thrombocytopenia.

  Other side effects can occur, including:

- sore mouth or throat or changes in taste and appetite
- peripheral neuropathy (nerve damage)
- changes in bowel habits, eg constipation or diarrhoea.

  Bladder irritation can occur. Your medical team might recommend that you drink 2 litres of fluid for 2 days following chemotherapy treatment to avoid it. They should tell you what to do if you have any symptoms of bladder irritation like burning, stinging or blood in your urine.

There are many less common side effects of chemotherapy, eg gout. Gout is a painful inflammation (redness and swelling) in your joints that can happen when cells are broken down rapidly during your first course of chemotherapy, leading to a build-up of uric acid in your joints.

NHS Choices have more information on gout.

30.2.2 Side effects of radiotherapy

The side effects of radiotherapy depend on the area of your body that is treated. For example, if you have radiotherapy to the head, neck or upper chest you may have a sore mouth or throat. Many people treated with radiotherapy have sore skin in the treated area.

30.2.3 Side effects of other treatments for lymphoma

Other treatments for lymphoma also can cause side effects. The most common side effects of these treatments are described within relevant pages:

- antibody therapy, rituximab
- newer, targeted treatments for lymphoma
- steroids
- radioimmunotherapy
- supportive treatments, which don't treat the lymphoma but support your body through treatment.

30.3 What should you do if you have side effects?

You are very likely to get side effects as part of your treatment, but try not to be discouraged. Side effects are usually temporary and often things can be done to make them easier to cope with.

Tell your medical team if you are having any side effects. You should also let them know if your side effects change during your treatment or don't get better. Unless you tell them, your medical team won't know how you are feeling.

There are treatments to help with many side effects. Some problems can be treated more effectively if they are caught early. Your medical team can also give you advice to help you cope with side effects.

31 Late effects of lymphoma treatment

Late effects are health problems that first appear months or years after treatment has finished. Most people recover well from treatment for lymphoma, but a few develop late effects. This page tells you about the potential late effects of lymphoma treatment. Detecting early signs of these late effects early can limit the problems they cause.

31.1 What are late effects?

Treatment for lymphoma nowadays is generally successful. Most people live for many years after their treatment has finished. Most people recover well from their treatment although some side effects can be long-term (take months or years to resolve) and a few may be permanent, such as reduced fertility.

Some people have health problems that first appear months or years after treatment has finished – these are known as '**late effects**'. You may hear people refer to these problems as having a 'delayed onset', which means they don't appear while you have treatment or immediately afterwards.

As people survive longer after their treatment for lymphoma, certain health concerns, like heart problems or second cancers, are slightly more likely to happen in people who had been treated for cancer than in the general population. However, there has often been a long time between treatment ending and the problem appearing.

It takes many years before doctors can know what late effects a treatment can have, if any. Modern lymphoma treatments are designed to limit the risks of future health problems. The treatments used today are expected to have a much lower risk of late effects than those we describe. However, this can only be confirmed after the treatments have been used for several years.

No treatment is without risk as it must be strong enough to treat the lymphoma successfully.

31.1.1 How to find out more about the risks of treatment

Before your treatment begins, talk to your medical team about both the short-term and long-term risks of your treatment plan. Your doctor's main concern is to treat your lymphoma successfully while minimising unwanted side effects.

As modern treatments are designed to reduce the risk of late effects as much as possible, fewer people should now be affected by health problems related to their lymphoma treatment. Research continues in order to understand how best to tailor treatments to each person to reduce the risk of long-term and late effects.

The risk of late effects may seem worrying, but being aware of potential problems gives you the best chance of successful treatment of any problems that occur.

There are some simple steps you can take to help look after yourself:

- Talk to your medical team about the risks of your treatment before it begins.
- Ask what symptoms you should look out for.

- See your doctor promptly if you have any concerns.

    You know your own body best. If you are worried about any symptoms you are having, talk to your medical team. If you have been discharged from lymphoma follow-up, see your GP. If you are still worried, you may wish to be referred back to your lymphoma team.

31.2 Who is at increased risk of late effects?

Your risk of late effects depends on a number of different factors, known as 'risk factors'.

Risk factors relate to the lymphoma you had, the treatment you had and individual factors:

- **Lymphoma-related risks**: the type of lymphoma you had, where it was growing and the organs and tissues it affected.
- **Treatment-related risks**: the specific drugs and types of treatment (eg chemotherapy or radiotherapy) you had, the dose and schedule of treatments, and how many different treatments you had.
- **Individual risks**: your age, any health problems you had before your treatment for lymphoma, your genes and family history as well as your lifestyle.

Having risk factors doesn't mean you will develop late effects. Many people have no late effects from their lymphoma treatment despite being at higher than average risk.

31.3 What are the potential late effects of lymphoma treatment?

The most common late effects that occur in people treated for lymphoma are described in relevant sections by type of treatment:

- late effects of chemotherapy
- late effects of radiotherapy
- late effects of newer, targeted therapies.

If you have been treated with a single type of therapy only, you might want to read only the section that applies to that type of treatment.

Some late effects aren't linked to a particular type of treatment. If you've had Hodgkin lymphoma, you are at an increased risk of developing non-Hodgkin lymphoma (NHL). It is not clear why this is.

31.4 What are the potential late effects of chemotherapy?

Different chemotherapy drugs have different potential late effects. Your doctor should give you more information about the exact drugs used in your treatment.

Cancer Research UK have information on the side effects of individual drugs used in cancer treatment.

31.4.1 Second cancers

If your lymphoma comes back after treatment, it is called a 'relapse'. If you develop a **different** type of cancer after treatment for lymphoma, this is called a 'second cancer'.

Chemotherapy can increase your risk of some types of cancer, particularly if you have high dose therapy.

Second cancers that have been linked to treatment with chemotherapy for lymphoma include:

- **Leukaemia** – particularly acute myeloid leukaemia (AML), which can develop on its own or after you have first developed myelodysplastic syndrome (MDS – where your bone marrow no longer makes enough healthy blood cells). If you would like more information about MDS, NHS Choices have an overview. You can find more information on AML from Cancer Research UK.
- **Lung cancer** – a small increase in the risk of lung cancer has been linked to some chemotherapy drugs grouped as 'alkylating agents', like mechlorethamine. This risk is much higher if you are a smoker and continue to smoke throughout and after your treatment.
- **Skin cancer** – some chemotherapy drugs can cause skin problems such as rashes and sensitivity to the sun. They can also increase your risk of skin cancer. Make sure you protect your skin from the sun. The British Association of Dermatologists have more information on what to look out for and how to protect yourself against skin cancer.

An increased risk of developing cancer usually persists for many years and second cancers are most likely to develop several years after your lymphoma treatment had finished.

Standard chemotherapy regimens (combinations of drugs) for Hodgkin lymphoma have changed in recent years. The ABVD chemotherapy regimen (combination of drugs) commonly used for Hodgkin lymphoma has a lower risk of causing a second cancer than regimens used in the past as it does not include alkylating agents.

31.4.2 Heart disease

Chemotherapy drugs called 'anthracyclines', like doxorubicin, may increase your risk of heart problems. They are part of many chemotherapy regimens used for lymphoma including CHOP and ABVD. It is well known that they can damage heart muscle, so that it can't pump strongly enough, but they work well for treating lymphoma. Your risk of heart problems increases with higher doses or more courses of treatment with anthracyclines.

Your doctors have to balance the possible risk of heart problems with giving you the most effective treatment for your lymphoma. You may also have tests to check that your heart is working effectively before you start treatment.

Heart problems become more common 10 years or more after your treatment but can occur sooner. Your risk of heart problems stays higher than usual for a number of years.

The British Heart Foundation have more information about heart problems. They also offer advice on keeping your heart healthy.

31.4.3 Lung problems

Some types of chemotherapy can cause damage to your lungs. The damage is a result of fibrosis (scarring).

One of the chemotherapy drugs that can cause lung problems is bleomycin. This drug is commonly used for Hodgkin lymphoma as part of the ABVD regimen.

Once it develops, lung fibrosis is usually permanent. If the damage is mild, it can be seen on X-rays or scans, but does not cause you any symptoms. More damage can cause symptoms like shortness of breath. If you are affected, you might not be able to do as much exercise as you used to.

If you have been treated with bleomycin and you need to have an operation in the future, you should tell the anaesthetist about it.

Doctors are looking at ways to reduce the risk of lung problems after treatment for lymphoma. Clinical trials of people with Hodgkin lymphoma suggest that bleomycin can be dropped for future cycles in some people who had a good response to their first 2 cycles of ABVD. In initial results from the trial, dropping bleomycin didn't affect the outcome for these people.

31.4.4 Other late effects of chemotherapy

There are some other uncommon late effects of chemotherapy.

Some types of chemotherapy, especially at high dose, could increase the risk of problems with your teeth if you don't look after them properly. Follow your dentist's advice to keep your teeth healthy.

The risk of developing eye problems, eg cataracts (cloudy patches in the lens of your eye that reduce your vision), is also higher if you have been treated with high doses of steroids. These are used alongside chemotherapy to treat some lymphomas. In certain people, steroids can also cause glaucoma. This can result in a loss of vision because of the build-up of pressure in the eye.

It is important that you visit your dentist and optician regularly.

What are the potential late effects of radiotherapy?

The potential late effects of radiotherapy depend greatly on what area of your body was treated. We describe the most common late effects of radiotherapy in the following sections. Your doctor should give you more information on the risks associated with your specific treatment plan.

31.4.5 Second cancers

If your lymphoma comes back after treatment, it is called a 'relapse'. If you develop a **different** type of cancer after treatment for lymphoma, this is called a 'second cancer'.

A higher risk of second cancer related to radiotherapy persists for at least 25 years after the start of treatment. Much of what is known about the risks of second cancers comes from older studies in people with Hodgkin lymphoma. People with Hodgkin lymphoma used to be treated with high doses of radiotherapy given to large areas of the body. Nowadays, smaller doses of radiotherapy are given in a more targeted way. However, researchers are unable to say for certain if these approaches are safer until they have been used for many years.

It is not as common for people treated for non-Hodgkin lymphoma (NHL) to have radiotherapy so there are fewer studies on its effects in people with NHL. However, if you've had radiotherapy as part of your treatment, the same advances in more precise targeting of smaller doses of radiotherapy apply to you, too.

The type of second cancer you are most at risk of depends on the area of your body that has been treated with radiotherapy. If you've had radiotherapy, ask your specialist what cancers you are at higher risk of developing. Make sure you know the symptoms of these cancers. Cancer is usually more treatable if diagnosed early.

If you've had **radiotherapy to the chest**, you are at increased risk of developing:

- breast cancer
- lung cancer
- cancer of the oesophagus (the tube leading from your mouth to your stomach).

Your risk of lung cancer is further increased if you smoke. Consider quitting to moderate this risk.

It is routine practice in the UK for women who were under 30 when treated with radiotherapy to the breast area to have breast cancer screening. This is because your risk of developing breast cancer is highest if you were under 25 when you received radiotherapy.

Screening is offered from the age of 30 or from 8 years after radiotherapy, whichever is later. Screening can detect breast cancer at an early stage, allowing the best chance of successful treatment.

NHS Choices has more information on breast cancer screening. You might also want to read the NHS's leaflet on screening for women at higher risk of breast cancer. Radiotherapy to other areas increases your risk of some types of cancer:

- **radiotherapy to the head and/or neck** increases your risk of head and neck cancers, including cancers of the mouth, tongue and thyroid gland

- **radiotherapy to the abdomen** (tummy) increases your risk of bowel cancer and other cancers of the digestive system, eg pancreatic cancer and stomach cancer.

You also have a higher risk of **skin cancer** in the area treated by radiotherapy. Protect your skin from the sun.

The British Association of Dermatologists have more information on what to look out for and how to protect yourself against skin cancer.

31.4.6 Heart disease and stroke

Radiotherapy to the chest can cause heart problems, including abnormal heart rhythms and damage to your heart valves or muscle. Hardening of your arteries can also happen. Radiotherapy to the neck might also cause hardening of your arteries. This can affect the blood supply to your brain, increasing your risk of stroke.

You may have tests to check that your heart is working effectively before you start treatment. Nevertheless, you may still develop heart problems after treatment. The risk of developing heart problems is increased with higher doses of radiotherapy. Your doctors have to balance the potential risk of heart problems in the long-term with giving you the most effective treatment for your lymphoma.

Heart problems become more common 10 years or more after treatment but can occur sooner. Your risk of heart problems stays higher than usual for many years. It is important that you are aware of this continuing risk and follow lifestyle advice to keep your heart healthy.

The British Heart Foundation have more information about types of heart problems. They also offer advice on keeping your heart healthy.

31.4.7 Thyroid problems

The thyroid gland produces hormones that regulate the speed at which the cells in your body work. It is found in the middle and front of the neck, so it is always exposed during radiotherapy to the neck. It is common for the thyroid gland to become underactive as a result. This is called 'hypothyroidism' and makes the cells in your body slow down. It can be diagnosed by a blood test.

You might feel tired a lot of the time and be more sensitive to cold. You could gain weight, too. These symptoms can be hard to detect and can be caused by other things. It is important that you know that these symptoms could be a sign of thyroid problems, so you can seek medical advice.

If your thyroid gland is affected by radiotherapy, problems might not develop for some years after you finish your treatment. The risk of developing hypothyroidism is higher in the first 5 years after treatment, but remains increased after that time.

You should be given regular thyroid function tests. Tell any doctors treating you that you've had treatment for lymphoma, so they are aware that you are at greater risk of thyroid problems. If you think you might be affected by thyroid problems and are no longer being followed-up by your lymphoma specialist, talk to your GP.

Tablets to replace thyroid hormones can correct hypothyroidism completely. You need to take these for the rest of your life.

There is also an increased risk of developing thyroid cancer many years after radiotherapy to the neck.

31.4.8 Effects on growth

Radiotherapy can affect the growth of bones and soft tissue in the area that has been treated. This is an important consideration in children and adolescents who are still growing. The effects on growth become apparent only several years after treatment. Our information for parents of children affected by lymphoma describes this and other late effects that might happen in children.

31.4.9 Other late effects of radiotherapy

Other possible late effects of radiotherapy include:

- **lung problems**: radiotherapy to the chest can cause damage to your lungs. The damage is a result of fibrosis (scarring).
- **dental problems**: radiotherapy to the head and neck can lead to an increased risk of tooth decay. Follow your dentist's advice to keep your teeth healthy.
- **eye problems**: if you've had radiotherapy to an area that includes the eyes, you might have dry eyes. Should this apply to you, there are treatments that can help. You are also at increased risk of developing cataracts (cloudy patches in the lens of your eye that reduce your vision) in the future.

31.5 What are the potential late effects of newer, targeted treatments?

There are many newer, targeted treatments being used for lymphoma. Scientists can only know for certain whether these treatments cause late effects many years after they have been in widespread use. However, so far, these treatments are generally expected to cause fewer side effects than chemotherapy and fewer late effects than other types of treatment, including chemotherapy and radiotherapy.

Research so far has shown that the new targeted drug brentuximab vedotin might contribute to lung damage, particularly if given in a regimen with bleomycin.

31.6 How can I reduce the risk of late effects?

Monitoring your health and how well you are recovering from treatment is an important part of your follow-up after treatment. Your medical team can advise you what you can do to reduce your risk of developing late effects and what to look out for. You can't always stop late effects from developing but catching problems early gives you the best chance of being treated successfully. If you have any health problems, talk to your medical team.

31.6.1 Be aware of your risks – look out for symptoms

- Find out what your risks are – ask your medical team exactly what treatment you've had and what your individual risks are. Keep this information in case you need it. Late effects can occur many years after treatment, when you might have been discharged from follow-up.
- Find out what symptoms you should be aware of.
- Ask what cancers you are at higher risk of developing and when the risk is highest – cancers are usually more treatable if diagnosed early. Make sure you know the symptoms of these cancers.

31.6.2 Monitor your health to find problems early

- Attend your follow-up appointments – monitoring and treatment of long-term and late effects is an important part of your follow-up after treatment. Make a note of any concerns to discuss at your appointments. Ask for your appointment to be brought forward if you are worried.

- Get to know what is normal for you – be aware of your body and how you usually feel. If you think something is not right, visit your GP or contact your lymphoma specialist.
- Have regular check-ups with your dentist and optician.
- Ask your lymphoma specialist or GP about cancer screening – screening programmes are specifically designed to find cancers early.

31.6.3 Follow a healthy lifestyle – give yourself the best chance of a healthy future

- eat a healthy diet and maintain a healthy weight
- exercise regularly
- give up smoking
- drink alcohol within recommended limits
- protect your skin from the sun.

Read our section on living with lymphoma for more information on how to look after yourself.

Macmillan Cancer Support and NHS England have set up the National Cancer Survivorship Initiative to help people live healthy and active lives with and beyond cancer. You can find out more from their website.

Tell any doctor looking after you about the treatment you have had for lymphoma. They need to be aware that you might be at increased risk of developing some health problems.

31.6.4 Research into reducing the risk of late effects

Treatment of lymphoma has changed over the years based on what doctors know about late effects. If you are being treated today, you should be at a lower risk of future health problems than people treated in the past. If you had treatment many years ago, understanding your risks now allows you and your doctors to monitor your health closely. Detecting problems early – including through formal screening programmes – means they are likely to be more easily dealt with.

32 Living with lymphoma

Living with and beyond lymphoma can be challenging. You may need to adjust to changes in your physical health, cope with difficult feelings, and deal with new challenges in your day-to-day life. Many people call this finding their 'new normal'.

32.1 Staying healthy

If you have, or have had, lymphoma, it is important to stay as healthy as you can. A healthy lifestyle can:

- help you enjoy your day-to-day life
- help your body cope better with any treatment you are having, or might need in the future
- lower your risk of developing serious illnesses in the future, including late effects (health problems that develop months or years after treatment has finished)
- help with your physical and emotional recovery.

Generally, the advice for staying healthy for someone affected by lymphoma is the same as it is for anyone else: eat a healthy diet and keep as active as you can. However, you may need to make some adjustments depending on your level of fitness and any side effects key worker about this even after you finish your treatment.

Remember to attend all your follow-up appointments and any regular routine health tests you're offered, such as checks for high blood pressure and screening for other cancers.

On these pages, you'll find information and advice on how to stay healthy when you have lymphoma:

- Diet and nutrition
- Exercise
- Stopping smoking
- Follow-up appointments
- Vaccinations
- What happens if lymphoma relapses (comes back)
- Palliative care (treatment to relieve symptoms)

32.2 Feelings

You may experience a whole range of feelings if you, or someone close to you, is living with lymphoma.

On these pages, you'll find information about some of the emotional issues you might face and tips on how to cope with them:

- The emotional impact of living with lymphoma
- Managing stress

32.3 Everyday life

Coping with everyday life can be stressful when you are already going through a difficult time. The effects of lymphoma and side effects of any treatment might also make everyday life more challenging than usual.

33 Self-management and remote monitoring

More and more people are living longer after a diagnosis of lymphoma. This has prompted some hospitals to change the way they organise long-term management and follow-up for people who have finished treatment for lymphoma.

33.1 Self-management

Most of the time, people make their own decisions about their health and wellbeing. When you have a long-term illness like lymphoma, it can feel as though many of those decisions are taken away from you.

Self-management involves taking control of your own health and wellbeing, even if you have a long-term condition. As well as your physical health, it includes taking an active role in managing your diet, exercise and emotional wellbeing.

Self-management is encouraged throughout your lymphoma care pathway, from diagnosis to treatment and beyond. It may become more formalised as you finish treatment and are offered the recovery package.

When you have a long-term illness like lymphoma, managing your own health can be daunting. This is why hospitals are developing self-management support pathways, which involve a combination of:

- personal support for you
- remote monitoring of your health.

33.2 Self-management support

Self-management support is a pathway that helps you develop the knowledge, confidence and skills you need to manage the physical, emotional and social impact of your lymphoma. It supports you to take an active role in your long-term care and to participate in health decisions with your medical team.

Self-management support is tailored to your individual needs. It aims to help you recognise and develop your own strengths and abilities so you can live an independent and meaningful life.

Although self-management support aims to put you in control, it's important to remember that you are **fully supported** by your lymphoma team throughout. Help and advice is always available if you need it. It is used together with remote monitoring to make sure you remain healthy.

Self-management support may also be called 'supported self-management'.

33.2.1 Why is self-management support used?

Self-management has a number of benefits for people with long-term conditions, such as lymphoma.

- It helps you achieve what's important to you.
- It can increase your self-confidence.
- It enables you to have meaningful discussions with your medical team.
- It can improve your quality of life.
- It gives you more sense of control over your life.

33.2.2 Who is self-management support for?

Self-management support is beneficial for anybody with a long-term health condition. Exactly what it involves depends on your individual needs.

Remember, self-management support does not mean you're on your own –you are supported to make decisions about your health and wellbeing. For people with lymphoma, it is used alongside remote monitoring or regular follow-up pathways so you can always access your medical team if you need to.

33.2.3 How does self-management support work?

When you finish treatment, you have a needs assessment as part of the recovery package. This is usually a simple questionnaire that you fill in either yourself or with a member of your medical team. The needs assessment helps identify your physical, practical, emotional and social needs. Your medical team can use it to create a care and support plan that's specific to you.

You should also be invited to a workshop on how to live healthily after treatment. This includes practical advice on staying fit and active, adjusting to life beyond cancer and coping with long-term effects. It also covers signs and symptoms to look out for and who to contact if you notice them. If you have not attended a wellbeing workshop, many charities offer free, local events, such as our Live your Life workshops or Macmillan's HOPE programme.

If you are going on a remote monitoring scheme, you also have a discussion with a member of your team, or attend a specific workshop, on how the system works and how and when you should contact your lymphoma team to arrange a follow-up appointment.

33.3 Remote monitoring

Remote monitoring goes hand-in-hand with self-management. It is a way for your medical team to keep an eye on your health without routinely seeing you face-to-face.

Instead of a traditional follow-up schedule where you have regular outpatient appointments with your medical team, remote monitoring involves booking your own follow-up appointments as-and-when you feel you need them – for example:

- if you notice any new or worsening symptoms
- if you are worried your lymphoma might have relapsed (come back)
- if you are struggling with long-term or late effects of lymphoma or its treatment
- if you are finding it hard to cope emotionally.

You might also hear this called 'patient-triggered follow-up'.

Although remote monitoring may seem daunting at first, you are fully supported by your lymphoma team throughout. You are given clear guidance on what to look out for and when to contact your medical team.

33.3.1 Why is remote monitoring used?

Although some people find regular follow-up appointments reassuring, many people feel very anxious in the days and weeks beforehand. Follow-up appointments are also time-consuming, sometimes involving several hours of travelling and waiting around for a short appointment. If you are feeling well, this can seem unnecessary.

Research has shown that if lymphoma relapses (comes back), it's usually noticed first by the person with lymphoma. Although it can be upsetting thinking about potential relapse, there is no evidence that regular follow-up appointments prevent relapse, pick-up relapses any earlier, or affect how long you might live.

Remote monitoring avoids the anxiety and inconvenience of regular follow-up and puts you in control – after all, you know what is normal for you and, with support, you will recognise when you need to be seen by your medical team.

Remote monitoring has a number of benefits:

- Any concerns can be dealt with quickly because you request an appointment as soon as you notice issues rather than waiting for a pre-booked appointment.
- You don't have to attend appointments when you feel well.
- You are actively involved in your recovery, which has the potential to improve your quality of life.
- You are less likely to need urgent appointments or emergency hospital admissions because you are better able to monitor and manage your own health needs.
- You get to take back some control over your life.

Remote monitoring may not be the right choice for everyone. You may have particular concerns or issues that make a traditional follow-up schedule more appropriate for you. Your medical team will discuss these with you.

33.3.2 Who is remote monitoring for?

Remote monitoring is suitable for people who are in full or partial remission and are at low risk of relapse. It is not offered at all hospitals so you may not be eligible even if you fit these criteria. It may not be suitable for you if you have had a stem cell transplant or had treatment as part of a clinical trial.

If you are worried about remote monitoring, tell your medical team. They can answer any questions you have. They consider your individual circumstances when planning your follow-up care and, in some cases, they may decide you are better suited to a traditional follow-up pathway.

Don't be concerned if you are not offered remote monitoring. There are lots of reasons that it may not be suitable for you. If you are worried, ask your medical team why they have recommended your particular follow-up plan.

33.3.3 How does remote monitoring work?

If you are on remote monitoring, you usually have regular blood tests to check your full blood count, liver, bone and kidney function, and any signs of inflammation. These are usually done at your GP surgery. Some people might have regular chest X-rays. The results should be sent to you and to your GP.

If your test results are normal, you are not given an automatic appointment with your hospital team. You can, however, request one whenever you have any concerns you'd like to discuss.

How long you are on remote monitoring for depends on several factors, including the type of lymphoma you have, your individual circumstances, and the usual practice at your hospital.

Some hospitals offer follow-up appointments on request indefinitely. Others discharge you if you remain well for a specified period, often 5 years. If you are discharged from remote monitoring, your GP becomes your main point of contact for any concerns you have. They can refer you back to your hospital team if necessary.

33.4 When to book an appointment

Your medical team will tell you the signs and symptoms of relapse (lymphoma coming back) or late effects to look out for before you start remote monitoring. Although it can be upsetting thinking about potential relapse, it is important to know what to look out for and to recognise if you need to book an appointment. Most people become more comfortable with these signs as they get used to being on remote monitoring.

If you notice any of these signs, or you have any concerns about your lymphoma, you can request an appointment.

You should contact your medical team to book a follow-up appointment if you have:

- enlarged lymph nodes lasting more than a week
- drenching night sweats
- unexplained weight loss
- worsening fatigue
- itching
- rashes (if you have a skin lymphoma)
- persistent or unexplained pain
- any new symptoms in any part of your body that last for more than 2 weeks

- any new or worsening side effects, possible side effects or late effects of your treatment
- difficulty coping emotionally or physically
- any other concerns relating to your lymphoma or your treatment (for example, fertilityconcerns).

33.5 Life on self-management and remote monitoring

Self-management gives you back responsibility for your own health. Although this has a lot of benefits, it can also be daunting, especially at first. You might feel anxious that you won't be attending regular appointments any more. It may take a while for your confidence to come back.

Remember that you are **fully supported** by your medical team at all times. They should make sure you have the information, skills and support you need to cope with the physical, social and emotional impact of lymphoma and to adjust to life after treatment. This may be written down in a personalised care plan as part of your recovery package. If you don't have one, or if there is anything you don't understand, ask your medical team.

When you are on remote monitoring, you can contact your medical team at any time.

Some people use diaries or apps, such as Macmillan's organiser, to track changes in symptoms or emotions. Other people use wearable technology to monitor their activity levels, sleep patterns, heart rate and blood pressure.

34 Lymphoma and the end of life

What you might experience in the final stages of life when you have advanced lymphoma. Please note that you may find this information distressing.

34.1 How do I know when to end active treatment?

Deciding to end active treatment is deeply emotional and personal. Although people close to you might offer their views, the final decision is between you and your medical team. In some cases, doctors may not be able to offer any further treatment. This might be because the lymphoma is not responding to treatment, or because you are not well enough to tolerate further treatment.

Throughout your treatment, you should be offered palliative care to maintain your quality of life. ('Palliative' comes from the word to 'palliate', which means to relieve or to lessen suffering.) If there is no further treatment for your lymphoma, your medical team should continue to offer you palliative care. The type of palliative care you receive depends on your needs and wishes. It often includes pain relief and symptom control. Your care should be holistic, which means that any physical, practical, social, emotional and spiritual needs you have are addressed.

There are many factors to consider when deciding whether to continue with active treatment for your lymphoma.

34.1.1 Is further treatment likely to work?

The treatment is less likely to work each time your lymphoma relapses (returns). The lymphoma cells can become resistant to treatment. This means that remission (reducing or ridding your lymphoma) might only last for a short time before you relapse again. Your doctors carefully consider whether further treatment is likely to work.

34.1.2 What are the risks of further active treatment?

Further treatment often means using stronger treatments. Unfortunately, as well as acting on the lymphoma, these treatments may pose significant health risks. Some treatments can be life-threatening if you are frail or have other health problems.

The side effects of stronger treatments can be severe. They might make you feel very unwell and stop you from enjoying the things that matter to you. Many people choose a better quality of life over a longer life. This means different things to different people, so it's important to think about your own priorities.

You and your medical team should weigh the potential risks and benefits of having further treatment. People often think about things they're looking forward to (eg a wedding). They base their decision on what is likely to help them feel as well as possible to enjoy the time they have left.

Deciding to stop active treatment does not mean that you are giving up. For many people, it is a choice to live their final days as comfortably and feeling as well as possible.

34.2 Can I enter a clinical trial?

When there is no further treatment for your lymphoma, you may wonder whether a clinical trial could benefit you. Clinical trials are medical research studies involving human volunteers. Clinical trials for lymphoma often test a new treatment, or how existing treatments could be used differently.

Only a small proportion of people with lymphoma are treated as part of a trial. There are lots of reasons for this. There are only a limited number of trials running at any time. Trials have strict eligibility criteria to make sure participants are safe and that the results are scientifically valid. There is not a suitable trial for everyone at any given time.

Finding out that there are no suitable trials can be distressing. You might feel that you have nothing to lose and wish to participate in a trial even if you do not meet its eligibility criteria. Please remember that your doctors cannot enter you into a trial unless you meet the criteria. Talk to your medical team about your options if there isn't a trial you can take part in.

34.3 How do I tell friends and family I'm no longer receiving active treatment?

It can be tough for the people around you to hear that you have decided to end active treatment. They might find your decision hard to accept and may try to change your mind. Be honest with them about your decision-making process so that they can see how you have reached your decision. If you wish, you could also ask your doctor to be with you to help explain. Although the conversation may be difficult, open communication can help to avoid misunderstandings and further distress.

34.4 How much time do I have left to live?

Your doctors may be able to give you an idea of how much time you can expect to live. They base this on the type of lymphoma you have, how fast it is growing and how it affects your vital organs (brain, heart, liver, kidneys and lungs).

Even with all this information, nobody can say for certain how long you have left. Many people choose to take a day at a time, enjoying the time they have left as much as possible.

34.5 How does lymphoma lead to the end of life?

There are a number of things that can happen to your body as you come towards the end of your life. Usually these changes happen because of the impact lymphoma has on your organs and the effects of advancing cancer on your body overall. Gradually, your body slows down and loses its function. Death from lymphoma is usually comfortable and peaceful.

When lymphoma involves a particular organ, it can stop that organ from doing its job. The problems you develop depend on which parts of your body have lymphoma involvement. We outline some possible changes to your body that you might experience in the final days of your life. Please remember it is difficult to predict exactly what will happen to you.

34.5.1 Bone marrow failure

Lymphoma often involves the bone marrow. Lymphoma can cause death when it affects the bone marrow to such an extent that you are unable to make new blood cells.

- Neutropenia: **shortage of white blood cells increases your risk of infection**. It is quite common for people with severe bone marrow disease to die from an infection (eg chest infection). Severe infection in 1 part of the body can lead to infection in the blood. When this happens, you might lose consciousness.

- Anaemia: **shortage of red blood cells prevents your organs from getting enough oxygen to function properly**. It can cause shortness of breath, weakness and fatigue.

- Thrombocytopenia: **shortage of platelets increases your risk of bleeding and bruising**. Bleeding can happen internally (inside your body, eg bleeding in your gut) as well as externally. Internal bleeding can cause serious complications and can be fatal. Thrombocytopenia may also increase your risk of bleeding in the brain, which can cause stroke.

To help you stay active and comfortable when your bone marrow is not functioning well, your doctors might offer you blood transfusions.

34.5.2 Chemical imbalance

You need a fine balance of salts and chemicals in your bloodstream to function properly. When you are well, your body regulates the levels, so that they are just right.

Advanced lymphoma can disrupt this fine balance. Tissues affected by lymphoma may produce abnormal levels of chemicals and waste products. Normally, the liver and kidneys cope with excess levels of chemicals by removing waste products. If lymphoma stops these organs from functioning as they should, it can lead to an imbalance of chemicals.

High levels of chemicals in the bloodstream often lead to a lower level of consciousness. You might feel confused, disoriented and drowsy. Your responses to things around you (such as noise, light and people around you) may become slow or stop entirely.

Increased salts and chemicals can also stop your organs from working properly. Hypercalcaemia (high levels of calcium in the blood) is a common problem for people with advanced cancer. It can lead to confusion and agitation. In some cases, it can stop your heart from beating regularly and lower your blood pressure.

34.5.3 Involvement of other organs

The symptoms you experience depend on which organs your lymphoma involves (affects).

If lymphoma involves your lungs, you are likely to have difficulties breathing. You also have an increased risk of chest infection, which can be difficult for your immune system to shake.

With liver involvement, the amount of healthy tissue in the liver progressively lessens. This stops your liver from doing important tasks such as: removing toxins from your blood; making the proteins needed to help blood clot; regulating your blood sugar levels; and producing bile, which is needed to digest food.

Liver disease can cause a range of problems, including:
- nausea (feeling or being sick)
- lowered appetite

- decreased levels of consciousness
- abdominal (stomach) swelling and discomfort
- jaundice (which makes your skin and the whites of your eyes look yellow)
- increased risk of bleeding
- fluctuating blood sugar levels.

Other organs may be affected by enlarged (swollen) lymph tissue pressing against them. As the tissue presses on your body tubes, it can cause blockages and pain. For example, pressure on the oesophagus (food pipe) can block the passage of food; pressure on blood vessels can block the passage of blood; pressure on the kidneys can block the passage of urine.

34.5.4 Hyperviscosity (thickness of blood)

'Viscosity' refers to the flow or thickness of blood. In advanced lymphoma, abnormal proteins produced by the lymphoma cells can cause hyperviscosity (thick blood). Dehydration worsens hyperviscosity.

If your blood is too thick, it can have difficulties passing through small blood vessels. This can lower the blood supply to organs such as your brain. When you don't get enough blood to your brain, you can have symptoms including:

- drowsiness or confusion
- headache
- blurred vision
- dizziness and
- loss of control over movements.

Hyperviscosity can also cause problems with the blood supply to your heart, making your heart beat irregularly.

34.5.5 Inability to close your eyes

As your muscles weaken towards the end of life, you may lose your ability to close your eyes. Your eyes may stay open even when you sleep. Should this happen, your eyes can be closed for you and gently lubricated to reduce dryness.

34.6 What symptoms might I have as I approach the end of life?

Your symptoms at the end of life depend on which of your organs are affected by lymphoma. You might also experience some of the more general symptoms. Your medical team can advise on how to cope with these symptoms.

34.6.1 Itching and sweats

Itching and drenching sweats (common symptoms of lymphoma) may worsen over time. You may be given a cream to alleviate the itching. To help with sweats, you might be given a fan and, in some cases, medication.

34.6.2 Weight loss

Weight loss can happen because the lymphoma is using up your energy supplies. Loss of appetite also often contributes to weight loss.

34.6.3 Loss of appetite

Losing your appetite is very common towards the end of life. Nutrition becomes less valuable to you as your body gradually loses the ability to absorb food and turn it into energy. As well as losing weight, you are likely to feel weaker and less able to concentrate. You may not want to eat or drink, especially if food makes you feel nauseous or if swallowing is painful.

If it is appropriate, your medical team may offer you special drinks and feeds. Your mouth may become dry because you are not drinking; if this is the case, your carers can help you stay comfortable by moistening your mouth and lips.

34.6.4 Fatigue and drowsiness

As you near the end of your life, you have less energy and need more rest. Even following or holding a conversation can be tiring.

Lymphoma uses a lot of your body's energy and resources. It can also stop your organs from getting the oxygen they need to function properly. This can lead to drowsiness and fatigue. In addition:

- chemical imbalances can lead to lowered levels of consciousness
- anaemia and infections can cause fatigue
- medication, eg pain relief or anti-anxiety tablets, may contribute to weakness and fatigue.

You are likely to become increasingly drowsy and spend more and more time sleeping. It might be difficult to wake you. In the final hours of your life, you may lose consciousness. You will probably continue to hear people around you and be able to feel their touch. Your loved ones can talk to you, be near to you and hold your hand.

34.6.5 Shortness of breath

Some people become short of breath or find it more difficult to breathe in the final weeks of life. This can be caused by anaemia limiting the amount of oxygen your tissues and organs get. To make up for this, you breathe harder.

Breathing difficulties can also be caused by lymphoma in the lungs, or the surrounding area. Your doctor can arrange for equipment (eg an oxygen cylinder) to help you breathe.

In the final days of your life, your breathing may become more noisy or irregular. This can happen because of the build-up of fluid in the throat. Your medical team can give you medication to help clear your throat. It can also happen as your throat muscles begin to relax.

34.6.6 Confusion and agitation

You may become confused and agitated as you approach the end of your life. There are various possible reasons for this, including chemical imbalances in the blood and the effects of certain medicines.

Your medical team should offer you medication and support to help you feel calmer, depending on why you feel confused or agitated.

Withdrawal and loss of interest

As your energy levels lower, you may lose interest in what is going on around you. Some people are less keen to see family and friends. You might find it easier to see an individual person at a time.

34.6.7 Circulation

Your blood circulation gradually slows down towards the end of life. When this happens, you are more sensitive to cold temperatures. Your hands and feet might feel cold. The skin on your face, hands, feet and legs might look pale, slightly blue and blotchy. Extra blankets or heat pads can help to keep you warm.

34.6.8 Incontinence (loss of bladder and bowel control)

You may lose control of your bladder and bowel. This is very common in the final stages of life. Your nurses may be able to provide pads to keep you comfortable and to protect your clothing and bed linen. Some people have a catheter fitted (a soft tube put into the bladder to drain urine away).

As you gradually eat and drink less, your body has less waste to remove. Incontinence becomes less of a problem. In the final hours of life, your kidneys stop making urine.

34.6.9 Pain

You may have pain in the last weeks of your life. Whether it happens depends on which areas of your body are affected by lymphoma and what damage it causes.

Your medical team should do all they can to lessen your pain. There are many medications they can offer, either on their own or in a combination. If a pain relief medicine is not effective, let a member of medical staff know, so they can try another. Morphine is the most common drug used to treat pain in cancer. It can also help with other problems, such as difficulty breathing.

34.6.10 How can my medical team help me?

Your medical team should offer you and your family support as you move towards the end of your life. They can provide information and answer questions. They can also offer pain relief and palliative care to help you to live comfortably in your final days.

The Department of Health (DoH) aims to support people in making decisions about their care and to end the variation in end of life care by 2020. They have recently published their key commitments, to:

- offer opportunities for honest discussions
- enable people to make informed decisions about their care
- provide personalised care plans for all
- allow discussion of personalised care plans
- involve family members and carers
- provide a main contact for people at the end of their life, available day and night.

34.7 How will I feel emotionally?

There is no 'normal' way to feel; the end of life is a very personal experience. How you feel depends on various factors. These might include your personality and outlook on life, your background, whether you are a religious or spiritual person, and how satisfied you feel with the life you have lived.

In 1969, Elizabeth Kübler-Ross, a Swiss psychiatrist, wrote a book called *On death and dying*. She spoke to over 200 people at the end of their life about how they felt. Kübler-Ross found that many people share common feelings and observed that these often occur in a pattern. Over the years, Kübler-Ross's ideas have received widespread support.

You might experience some, or perhaps all, of the following feelings. They don't have to occur in any particular order.

If you are close to someone who is dying, you are likely to experience a range of powerful emotions too. You may move back and forth between them, or skip some entirely. Some days, you might have several emotions all at once, which can feel overwhelming.

34.7.1 Shock

Even if you have had lymphoma for a long time and you know your treatment has not worked, it can still be a shock to hear that you will die from your illness. You may feel bewildered and unable to take information in. You might feel numb at first and feel very little. People around you may say that you seem very calm. Some people busy themselves with making practical arrangements when they are in shock, rather than considering how they feel emotionally.

34.7.2 Denial

Denial is very common. You may refuse to accept that you will soon die. However, you may be processing this information at a deeper level of consciousness. For example, you might talk about going on holiday next year, but make no booking arrangements.

Regardless of how many people are around you, you are likely to feel isolated. You might push away the people who are close to you while you try to deny what is happening.

Denial can be a useful defence to protect you from feeling emotionally pained and overwhelmed. It can help you to enjoy today without worrying about the future. However, it can also make it difficult for you and others to make preparations or to talk about things that are important.

Denial is not a state to be rushed or 'snapped' out of; you move beyond it when you are ready.

34.7.3 Anger

Anger is a common response to anxiety, fear and loss. As well as feeling angry about the impending loss of your life, you might feel angry about other things that have happened in the past. You might feel envious of the people around you who will continue to live after you die, for example family members and health professionals.

34.7.4 Bargaining

Some people try to strike bargains with a higher power, such as a god or the universe. This can take the form of 'deals' e.g., 'if you let me recover, I will lead a healthy life'. Similarly, some people have 'if only' thoughts e.g. 'if only I'd gone to the doctor sooner, I might not be in this situation'. These thoughts can be a way of trying to take control over a situation that is, ultimately, beyond anyone's control.

34.7.5 Grief and sadness

In Western cultures, grief and deep sadness are strongly associated with death. You are likely to experience these emotions for yourself as well as for loved ones. Sadness is natural as you approach the end of life. It can help you accept your situation. Some people might also have episodes of depression.

Conclusion

In the future, chemotherapy will no longer be necessary in the management of Hodgkin lymphoma. The utilisation of immunotherapy and novel combinations the side effects associated with chemotherapy can be avoided. The treatment of Hodgkin lymphoma has majorly impacted the care of patients with other types of cancer. Furthermore, there are higher cure rate in this disease represents one of the biggest victories in medical and radiation oncology. Moving forward, interim imaging and the frontline administration of novel agents will continue to enhance the treatment paradigm. Given this success, a new course has been forged in survivorship care, as patients are now living for decades after their initial diagnosis. The goal in Hodgkin lymphoma is to cure patients with the least amount of treatment. However, if a patient progresses on all standard treatments it is appropriate to administer the older Mustargen Oncovin Procarbazine Prednisone (MOPP) chemotherapy regimen.

www.ingramcontent.com/pod-product-compliance
Lightning Source LLC
Chambersburg PA
CBHW031606210526
45464CB00004B/1445